W0259750

This intimate story tells of the Hagas' love of God as well as their devotion to each other, depicts the bravery of the cancer journey, the hope for a cure, and demonstrates what faith really is. Words can't express how deeply affected I was by reading *His Love Carries Me.* Following along on this remarkable quest, I could feel the moments with them, and I witnessed their love of God in every account. The author shares heartfelt, raw emotions that are known only to people experiencing a health crisis such as cancer. This should be a required read for all healthcare providers.

—Anne M., RN, BSN, Senior Research Nurse
Thoracic Head & Neck Medical Oncology
MD Anderson Cancer Center

His Love Carries Me is a unique perspective on health, sickness, love, and God through the eyes of a loving caregiver. The Hagas' journey with God captures the limitations of modern medicine, describes the day-to-day fight for healing, and provides a powerful example of one family's struggle to fight a menacing disease. After more than a decade in oncology, I learned a new aspect to my work with each chapter. Reading this captivating book helped me understand unwavering faith and will give encouragement to patients, caregivers, and healthcare providers alike. A must-read for everyone.

—Martin Frederik Dietrich, MD, PhD
Florida Hospital Cancer Institute
Orlando, FL

His Love Carries Me is an exceptional testimony of not only one family's faith, but of God's unwavering, steadfast faithfulness and grace. DeLayne Haga nails what it feels like to struggle through every step of a devastating diagnosis and bears her heart in this very personal and detailed account. This book will prove to be an invaluable resource for caregivers of persons with any illness. I highly recommend this boldly honest read along with its companion book of her late husband's spiritual journey, *Cancer on Two Wheels*. You won't be disappointed.

—Kristi Brashier

Written for caregivers of terminally ill patients, *His Love Carries Me* has a broader appeal as a gripping love story between a man, a woman, and God. DeLayne Haga takes readers on a roller coaster ride of emotions through sickness and health that will inspire readers to hang tightly to their faith. If anyone ever needed a good reason to hug her husband—and God—this book has that, and more.

—Lee Ann Bandy

DeLayne Haga's *His Love Carries Me* is a powerful story of her family's journey through lung cancer. God used her husband's diagnosis and treatment path, as well as DeLayne's caregiving experiences, to reach people and shape lives in sometimes surprising ways. I was encouraged to see how God provided and carried them through, shining His love in darkness and in light. I'd recommend this book not only to those who face a similar path, but also to anyone who hungers to see the ways God works in the lives of His people.

—Beth Mull

His *Love* Carries Me

A CAREGIVER'S STORY OF
FAITH, HOPE, & LOVE

DeLayne Haga

Carpenter's Son Publishing

His Love Carries Me

Published by Carpenter's Son Publishing, Franklin, Tennessee

Published in association with Larry Carpenter of Christian Book Services, LLC
www.christianbookservices.com

Published in association with Roaring Lambs Publishing, Dallas, Texas

Senior Editor: Tammy Kling

Assistant Editors: Tiarra Tompkins, Kristi Brashier, Lee Ann Bandy, and Beth Mull

Copy Editors: Christy Callahan, Kristi Brashier, and Lee Ann Bandy

Cover and Interior Design: Suzanne Lawing

Printed in the United States of America

ISBN 978-1-946889-61-4

Disclaimers: This memoir is based on actual events that occurred. Conversations come from the author's recollections and are not written to represent word-for-word transcripts. The essence of the dialogue and incidents are based on memory, journal entries, and medical records. This book is not intended as a substitute for the medical advice of physicians. The reader should consult a physician in matters relating to his/her health and particularly with respect to any symptoms that may require diagnosis or medical attention. In an effort to protect the privacy of individuals and businesses mentioned in this book, some fictional names are used and are denoted by an asterisk (*).

To my husband, Chris, who lived for me

To my Lord, Jesus Christ, who died for me

Your love carries me

CONTENTS

INTRODUCTION

In 2010, the love of my life was diagnosed with stage IV lung cancer that had metastasized to his brain. I was stunned—*he had never smoked.*

The mass in my husband's lung almost tripled in size within three months of diagnosis to 13 centimeters—almost half the length of a ruler—before we found a successful regimen to shrink the cancer. The doctor originally gave Chris a prognosis of six months. Instead, he lived six *years*. Because he was officially declared to have "no evidence of disease" on three separate occasions, I still refer to him as "My Miracle Man." I witnessed God's glory multiple times.

Amazingly, he worked full time throughout most of his treatment. He was even able to continue riding his bicycle for several years with a collapsed lung.

When asked to share what we had learned about living with this horrible disease, we became mentors to other lung cancer patients and their caregivers. We never turned down a request. God dealt us this hand for a reason, and we intended to make the best of a dreadful situation.

Our lives began reflecting the following scripture:

> *Praise be to the God and Father of our Lord Jesus Christ, the Father of compassion and the God of all comfort, who comforts us in all our troubles, so that we can comfort those in any trouble with the comfort we ourselves have received from God.*
>
> —2 Corinthians 1:3–4 NIV

My husband chronicled his spiritual journey in an inspirational blog. After his death in 2016, I decided to publish his works in *Cancer on Two Wheels—A Spiritual Journey with Stage IV Lung Cancer* as a tribute to his memory and to carry on his legacy of faith through trials. Because of the challenges I tackled head-on as Chris's advocate, others suggested I write a companion book to help patients as well as their caregivers, family, and friends affected by a devastating diagnosis. It helps to know you're not alone with what you're going through.

While getting ready for bed one night several months after Chris passed away, I thought of reasons why I couldn't write a book.

I'm not a writer and have never had a desire to write a book. I don't have a clue how to get a book published. I wouldn't even know what to title a book.

By the time I pulled down the bed covers, I had dismissed the idea of becoming an author. But as soon as my head hit the pillow, I heard a voice softly whisper, *His Love Carries Me.*

I sat straight up in bed. Tears filled my eyes as I realized God had just clearly spoken to me. The title was perfect. That's exactly how I coped with Chris's disease and how I was getting through my grief.

Over the next few weeks, it was challenging to focus on anything else. The Lord was nudging me to do something out of my realm of experience, and it was exciting. With Him leading the way, it appeared I would be writing a book after all.

My grief was still fairly raw, but I found myself smiling a lot as I wrote—much more than the crying you might expect. Reminiscing about times shared with the love of my life, both happy and poignant memories, keeps Chris close to my heart.

This book shares our experiences through my eyes as Chris's caregiver and advocate, filling in the blanks in his story along the way. It chronicles our spiritual and emotional journey, the search for an effective treatment, the problems we encountered along the way, our plans for the ominous what-if scenarios, and how God worked through a seemingly impossible situation.

Each cancer journey is unique and has its own issues and challenges to face. Hopefully, our experiences will help you advocate in any medical situation and encourage you to be proactive when facing life's adversities. Faith, hope, and love play an important role in winning the battle in any crisis. I pray you'll find strength through your faith as you experience trials of your own.

As you read this book, keep in mind this isn't just our story—it's God's story. We didn't walk this road alone, and you don't have to either.

I can do all things through Him who strengthens me.

—PHILIPPIANS 4:13

Chapter 1

MY FAITH TESTED

I had a relatively easy life up to the age of forty-nine, while so many people around me had major problems. I knew God allows adversity in people's lives for a number of reasons, but not because He doesn't love them. I also knew that when times are the toughest is when it takes the greatest faith. Untested faith requires no faith at all. I occasionally wondered, *When will the inevitable rock my world? Is my faith genuine? If my faith is tested, will I praise the Lord in both good times and bad?*

Chris, our sons, and I spent Christmas 2009 at my parents' home in Broken Arrow, Oklahoma. After we went to bed, I heard my dad coughing extremely hard in the bedroom across the hallway. He had been diagnosed with pulmonary fibrosis four years earlier, and I could see and hear his health rapidly declining. I feared he had just seen his last Christmas.

Worrying about my dad, I sobbed inconsolably.

Dad's health took a turn for the worse in March. The doctors gave him less than two weeks to live.

While Dad was in the hospital, my family grew fond of his nurses. We discussed who was our favorite, but we all picked someone different because they were all good. I decided to ask Dad his opinion.

"Who's *your* favorite nurse, Dad?"

Without hesitation, he turned his head, opened his eyes, and smiled at me. "You are." My heart melted. I'm glad he immediately closed his eyes again so he couldn't see me weeping.

My father died on March 30, 2010. It was an answer to prayers because of his poor quality of life. Both my family and I thought I would fall apart when Dad died because I was a "Daddy's girl." But knowing there's no more pain or suffering in heaven gave me unimaginable peace.

> *"There will be no more death or mourning or crying or pain, for the old order of things has passed away."*
>
> —REVELATION 21:4 NIV

At that time, Chris was riding his bike about eighty miles per week for exercise, trying to lose 5 pounds from his 195-pound frame. After several months of trying with no success, the weight was finally coming off fast. He lost 10 pounds. In late April, he developed a little cough with a tickle in his throat and chest while he was on a twenty-mile bike ride out in the country. He assumed it was just allergies.

The cough worsened, so Chris went to a doctor on May 10. He was diagnosed with an upper respiratory infection and given an antibiotic. His cough still didn't improve, so he saw our family physician on May 24. An x-ray showed pneumonia. The doctor prescribed a different antibiotic and an inhaler. Chris went back ten days later, still coughing.

The doctor listened to his lungs. "A lingering cough is normal after pneumonia," he said, "but your lungs sound clear."

I noticed Chris napped a lot, falling asleep just a few minutes after sitting down to watch television. That wasn't his norm. Unable to fall asleep one night, I went over his symptoms in my head. *A cough that doesn't go away, persistent pneumonia, constant fatigue, and sudden weight loss. Those are all symptoms of lung cancer. Nah, it couldn't be that—he's never smoked.* I dismissed the thought because our family doctor didn't suspect the disease.

On July 5, Chris felt better than he had in a long time and went on an eighteen-mile bike ride. He thought he was finally getting over the pneumonia, even though coughing harder. At my insistence, he reluctantly called his doctor that morning and saw him the same day. Another x-ray showed the pneumonia was actually worse. Baffled, his general practitioner referred him to a local pulmonologist. A week later, the pulmonologist ordered a third set of x-rays, which showed the pneumonia continued to worsen. He ordered a CT scan to see if he could determine the cause.

On July 15, 2010, I walked in the door from work, and my world changed in an instant. Chris stood in the kitchen at the edge of the counter.

"The doctor called me on the way home from work with the results of the CT scan."

"What did it show?" I asked, not at all suspecting what I was about to hear.

His chin quivered. "I have two tumors in my right lung."

I immediately thought of actress Dana Reeve, the widow of *Superman* actor Christopher Reeve. She was diagnosed with stage IV lung cancer in 2005 and died seven months later. She claimed she had never smoked, but I didn't believe her. Everyone "knows" that only smokers get lung cancer. I believed her now.

My legs felt weak and started to shake. I held Chris in my arms, embracing him silently for a long time as I let him cry. Reeling from the painful news, I was momentarily frozen in shock. I didn't shed a tear.

"We'll get through this," was all I could mutter, trying to be strong for him.

Then I wobbled into the bathroom on rubbery legs, closed the door, and bawled. As reality set in and my emotions thawed, terror seized me. *I don't want to be a widow! I'm too young to be a widow! I'm not ready to be a widow!* I silently screamed to God. In my anguish, I couldn't form a prayer.

I never heard of anyone surviving stage IV lung cancer for long, and I had no hope that the love of my life would. But God had a plan for the trial we faced.

> *In this you greatly rejoice, though now for a little while you may have had to suffer grief in all kinds of trials. These have come so that your faith—of greater worth than gold, which perishes even though refined by fire—may be proved genuine and may result in praise, glory and honor when Jesus Christ is revealed.*
>
> —1 Peter 1:6–7 NIV

Chapter 2

MR. RIGHT

"He's the one you'll marry," my mother said after I told her about my first date with Chris.

"What makes you think that? We've only gone on one date."

"You talk about him differently than other guys you've dated."

Mom was so sure of her intuition that a month later she bought wedding decorations. I thought she was jumping the gun, but I now see from my old diary entries I was falling in love with Chris from the very beginning.

When I attended Oklahoma State University in Stillwater, I dated several guys, but no one warranted a second date—until I met Rick, an engineering major, who reminded me of Tom Selleck in the *Magnum, P.I.* television show. Besides being attractive, intelligent, and funny, he was a Christian and a gentleman—my basic qualifications for a husband. I thought he was Mr. Right, but the feeling wasn't mutual. Although we dated some, we were just good friends who ran around with the same group. I was heartbroken when he didn't stay in touch after he graduated. I clung to the hope that someday he would come to his senses and realize I was the woman for him.

I didn't think to ask God to lead me to the man He had in mind for me. I assumed I could find a husband on my own.

I worked part time during college for PROCESS, a small word processing company started by a couple in their tiny home. Before I graduated in 1982, business was growing, and the owners offered me a full-time job. I agonized over the career decision. I didn't want to continue working for a small company, though I loved the work. Instead of praying, I asked my dad for his advice. Even though I failed to ask for guidance from my heavenly Father, God looked out for me. I accepted the offer.

Chris worked for one of our clients—the local newspaper, *Stillwater News Press.* He developed software for their circulation department and used our computer occasionally. I met him one day in my new temporary two-person office in a small building near downtown. We introduced ourselves, and then I went right to work, sitting at my desk with my back to him. After I found out he was a junior in college, I assumed he was younger and immature. I had graduated, was twenty-two, and considered myself a mature adult. Chris looked like an eighteen-year-old version of Opie Taylor from Mayberry. Little did I know, he was actually six months older than me and was working full time to put himself through college to get his engineering degree.

"I'm trying to cram my four-year degree into seven years," he joked with me later.

Eventually, my office moved just a few blocks from the *News Press.* Chris came by occasionally to drop off work. We never exchanged more than a "Hi, how are you?" Gary and Carole, the company owners, occasionally talked about what a nice guy Chris was and tried, but failed, to pique my interest in him. My heart was still set on Rick.

OUR FIRST DATE

I vividly remember stopping abruptly in the hallway of my apartment one morning in early July 1983. It suddenly dawned on me that God must not think Rick was Mr. Right.

"God, I haven't been able to find Mr. Right on my own. I'm leaving it up to You to bring him into my life, but please let our paths cross soon," I said audibly.

Although I had been a believer as long as I could remember and was baptized in the fifth grade, that's the first time I remember giving Him control of my life. I was about to learn a valuable lesson. God hadn't been refusing to answer my wishes for Mr. Right. He was simply saying, *Wait. I have someone better for you.* Sometimes the best things are appreciated more when we have to wait for them.

Two weeks later, Chris bought a new car and drove it to our office to give my boss a ride. When they got back, Gary turned to Chris.

"You ought to show DeLayne your car."

Was this a set-up?

I went with Chris to look at his sporty 1983 Dodge Shelby. I admired the car as we sat inside with the doors open.

"Would you like to go for a ride?" he asked.

"I guess we could take a spin around the block."

I was impressed with the car and suddenly wanted to know more about Chris. On the way back to the office, he casually asked me for a date.

"Would you like to go out to eat sometime?"

I eagerly accepted.

Although I didn't realize it then, God had quickly answered my prayer for Mr. Right. He'd been right under my nose for a year. If only I had opened my eyes, I would have recognized him.

Our first date was at a steakhouse. Both of us were introverts by nature, but we talked nonstop the entire evening. A Christian, Chris attended a small Bible church with his parents. His eyes lit up as he told me about his family. I was glad to learn he had a close relationship with his parents and siblings. Mom always said you can tell what type of husband a man will be by the way he treats his mother. When Chris told me he accidentally fractured his mother's ribs once because he hugged her too hard, I knew he must have a good relationship with her.

He looked up to his older brother, Randy, who had married his wife, Molly, just one month earlier. I was surprised Chris talked so much about their wedding. Most guys would shy away from the topic of marriage—especially on the first date. But not Chris. He even mentioned he wanted to get married someday, but he wasn't in any rush.

Since it was a beautiful summer evening and neither of us enjoyed the college-town nightlife, we drove to a kiddie park. Sitting on the swings, we talked until late in the night. I saw why everyone had wanted us to date—our lifestyles and personalities were compatible, and we were a good intellectual fit. Under his boyish appearance, he was handsome, but I was even more impressed with his integrity and work ethic, sense of humor, and quick wit. He imitated Steve Martin's version of "Mack the Knife," and I saw a playful side I hadn't expected.

"I've noticed Carole has started saying nice things about you and is having me relay messages to you rather than calling you herself," I said. "I think she's trying to get us together."

"Anita from the *News Press* has been *your* biggest cheering section. She has been pestering me for a year to ask you out. I wasn't sure you were available because of the diamond ring on your right hand."

The solitaire was a family heirloom from my great-grandmother.

Even though we were in a kiddie park, it was so peaceful and romantic there. We felt so comfortable around each other I didn't want the night to end. It was 11:30 before we realized it, and we had to be at work early the next morning.

"Do you have time to come in?" I asked when he drove me home.

"Yes," he answered, without hesitation.

Chris sat near the end of my long couch while I made tea. Then came the first awkward moment of the night—I didn't know where to sit. If I sat in the chair or at the far end of the sofa, I'd look unfriendly. If I sat right next to him, I might seem forward. I took my chances and squeezed in between Chris and the small space between him and the end of the couch.

He did most of the talking. I was so sleepy by then, my brain and mouth wouldn't coordinate.

"It's getting late. I'd better go," he said.

But he kept on talking. An hour later, he said for the third time, "I'd better go." He moved to face me and laid his right arm across the back of the couch behind me. I assumed he was getting ready to lean over and kiss me for the first time. We looked in each other's eyes.

Our second awkward moment. No kiss. I didn't want to just sit there as if I expected it, so I got up. He followed me to the door. As I opened it for him, Chris turned around, pulled me close, and tenderly kissed me as I wrapped my arm around his waist. I had tingles down to my toes as we embraced. I closed the door behind him, my heart pounding. I couldn't wait to see him again.

FALLING IN LOVE

Chris was on the *News Press* softball team, so I watched them play a few nights later. Afterward, we strolled hand in hand along the shore of Boomer Lake. We talked about how the two of us would be a hot topic now that everyone at the *News Press* knew we were dating. We wondered how long it would take Gary and Carole to find out. Over the next month, it became a game to see how long we could keep it a secret from them.

"Two years from now, I'd like to confess to Gary and Carole that we're dating and see their reaction," I said.

Chris smiled. "If we're still together in two years, we probably won't be 'just dating.' "

Love bloomed. The more we were together, the more we wanted to be with each other. Working full time and going to college took up most of Chris's day. By the time he finished his homework at my apartment, it didn't leave much quality time. He left my apartment at 2:30 a.m. sometimes, and I had to get up at 6:30 to get ready for work. We were zombies, but we were smitten.

A month passed, and my bosses still didn't have a clue we were dating. Chris called my office and spoke with Carole. After they hung up, Carole told me, "That was Chris . . . Haga . . . from the *News Press*" as if I didn't know who Chris Haga was. "He's such a nice guy, and he's so easy to work with."

I could barely contain my smile. *If only she knew.*

One evening Chris asked if I'd like to go for a drive. I could tell he had something on his mind. We ended up at a playground in the neighborhood where he grew up. Walking hand in hand, he led me to a bench, where we sat in the moonlight.

"My feelings for you are growing deeper and deeper and are getting past the 'caring for' stage. I'm starting to really love you," he said. "I'm starting to look down the road more and hope that the future will find us together."

I melted at the way he looked at me. But I wasn't ready to tell him I loved him, so I just smiled. Fortunately, he didn't give up on me.

THE ENTIRE PACKAGE

I found more and more things about Chris I admired. I mentioned to him that I never heard him cuss.

"You never will, if I can help it," he said. "I have too much respect for you."

He was true to his word. I only heard him cuss twice in the thirty-three years we were together—once when he started running a high fever for the umpteenth time, requiring another trip to the hospital, and the other was just a few weeks before he passed away.

My esteem grew when Chris told me he had strict moral values. He felt he owed it to his parents, himself, and to the Lord to stick to his values. I saw the way he interacted with his family, my family, co-workers, and friends. Everyone loved and respected him. I wrote a checklist in my diary of things I liked about Chris: same Christian beliefs, gentleman, doesn't cuss, doesn't smoke, doesn't drink alcohol, nice looking, intelligent, sensitive, good sense of humor, plus so much more.

He was the entire package—everything I wanted in a husband. We occasionally brought up the topic of marriage in general but were testing the waters to see if we were on the same page. Everyone else around us could see how perfect we were for each other and how happy we were together. They kept trying to rush us into getting married.

In early October, my employers discussed hiring Chris to work for them. When my parents came to visit for dinner, we talked about how his working there might affect our job performance.

"Some companies don't permit spouses working together," Mom said.

Chris almost choked when she referred to us as "spouses." And yet Gary and Carole were still clueless.

THE JOKE

A few weeks later, my company started selling computers with the software Chris had developed. Their newspaper ad included a photo of me sitting at a computer. The ad read, "Available at PROCESS," and it gave the phone number. We also gave pencil holders shaped like desktop computers to customers. The holders had a slot in the monitor to insert a photograph. Chris inserted my picture from the ad and put it on his desk.

After the advertisement appeared, I received a bouquet of red roses at the office. The card said, "Nice ad, but are you really available?" It was signed, "Your Secret Admirer." Carole asked who they were from.

"I don't know."

"Come on now—use your imagination," Carole said. "It's probably Chris at the *News Press*."

I turned around so she couldn't see the smirk on my face.

Two days later, Gary went to the *News Press* to talk with Chris about business. The receptionist asked Gary if she could have a pencil holder like the one on Chris's desk. Gary glanced at the pencil holder and did a double take when he saw my photo. Even though he was always quick to let people know how smart he was, he still hadn't realized we were dating.

"Chris, have you seen any florists lately?"

"C'mon, Gary, don't you know what's going on around you? We've been dating for three months."

MY REALIZATION

People speculated we would be engaged by Christmas and married within a year.

I spent Christmas in Oklahoma with my family while Chris and his family went to Louisiana. During my long drive back to Stillwater after the holiday, I pondered my relationship with Chris, realizing for the first time how deeply I loved him. I was ready to spend the rest of my life with him. Now I just had to wait for him to propose.

THE RINGS

In January, I dropped off two family heirloom diamond rings at a jeweler's to have them appraised. While working in Carole's office, I accidentally left a reminder note to myself on her desk, written in shorthand. "Call Gem Gallery on Friday to check on rings."

After work, I remembered the note. *Should I go back to the office and get it?* She could read shorthand. Suddenly, I felt mischievous.

Nope—I'll let her wonder.

The next morning, Carole laid the note on my desk without saying a word. However, she apparently had mentioned the note to her husband. That afternoon, I went into to Gary's office and asked if he had made arrangements yet for us to tour the *News Press.*

"No, my contacts there aren't as good as yours. By the way, how *is* Chris?"

Innocently, I shrugged my shoulders. "Ask him."

Gary grinned. "I think I can figure it out. You've had a glint in your eye lately."

Laughing, I started walking toward my office.

Gary called out to me as I walked down the hall, "Don't forget, you're not the only one around here who knows shorthand!"

Got him again!

AS ONE

In March of 1984, Chris and I began talking about marriage in earnest. One evening in my apartment, we discussed our finances to see if we could afford it. I showed Chris the handwritten ledger I kept of my monthly income and expenses. I guess he was impressed with my attention to detail and my ability to handle finances. He became strangely silent. Gently grabbing hold of my hand, he looked at me. His eyes sparkled.

"Will you marry me?"

"Are you serious?" I asked cautiously.

"Yes." He nodded.

Finally—the moment I had been waiting for. I was dying to accept, but there was one thing missing for this old-fashioned, sentimental gal.

"Then you need to get down on one knee."

He laughed. I smiled too, but I was serious. He complied and asked again. I eagerly accepted. It wasn't the most romantic proposal, but it got the job done. We decided to get married that summer between semesters—just three months later.

The church ceremony was beautiful. I wore a white gown with a long train and veil like I had dreamed of since I was a little girl. Dad walked me down the aisle to give my hand in marriage, both of us smiling from ear to ear. My parents were as excited to have Chris for a son-in-law as I was to have him as my husband. Chris stood at the end of the aisle, handsome in his black tuxedo. Filled with joy, I thought I might burst.

Because our relationship was built on a foundation of admiration for each other and mutual respect, I had married a man who had truly become my best friend. It was a strong base that kept our marriage resilient. As one, our relationship grew more beautiful through the test of time and the trials of life that lay far ahead.

FAMILY MAN

We moved to Midland, Texas, in 1985, and both of us worked for Texas Instruments. It was hard to leave our families behind in Oklahoma, but Chris and I realized later that being so far away from family and friends strengthened our marriage, since we had only ourselves and the Lord to rely on.

Our first son, Chad, was born three years later. In 1990, we transferred to Texas Instruments in Sherman, Texas. Shane was born the following year. Chris earned his MBA (Master of Business Administration) in 1995 and transferred two years later to the corporate office in Dallas. We relocated to McKinney so he could have a shorter commute. I quit my job and started a secretarial business at home so I could be with our boys as much as possible.

Chris was totally involved in our sons' lives from the day they were born. They were his pride and joy, and they adored him. A doting father, he felt his family was more important than climbing the corporate ladder. He loved to wrestle with the boys, and they always enjoyed being close to him.

Whatever Chad and Shane were interested in, so was Chris. He was a leader in the church's AWANA program, which helps children memorize Bible verses. He attended our sons' music recitals and concerts. He even taught them a little of his leatherworking hobby, helping them carve designs on wallets. He attended every soccer game, flag football game, and Tae Kwon Do event. Chris helped coach their basketball teams in elementary school, and he coached their baseball teams from Little League through middle school. Never pushy or expecting perfection, he simply encouraged them to always do their best and to pursue their interests.

When our sons took up competitive bicycling in their teen years, Chris began riding with them on their training rides. This allowed him to spend more time with them, get exercise, and make sure they were safe. We were spending so much time at races and money on cycling equipment that Chris turned his photography hobby into a part-time business venture and began photographing high school and collegiate races, since we would be there anyway.

He knew what a strong influence a father is in a boy's life because of the influence his own father had on him. Chris was a wonderful role model of how to treat a woman, whether it was his mother, his wife, a teacher, a nurse, a hotel maid, or a waitress. Our boys saw their dad reading his Bible every morning. His actions spoke louder than any words.

Train a child in the way he should go, and when he is old he will not turn from it.

—Proverbs 22:6 NIV

Chapter 3

OFFICIAL DIAGNOSIS

Without warning, lung cancer invaded our lives. We had the CT scan results but didn't know if the tumors were malignant. On July 21, 2010, Chris had a biopsy at our local hospital via a bronchoscopy, a procedure in which an instrument called a bronchoscope is threaded through the nose and down the throat to the lungs.

The doctor handed the CT scan report to me for our records before going with my husband to the operating room. Although I had no medical background whatsoever, I was able to figure out the right middle lobe was collapsed, and one mass appeared to be at least 5.7 cm by 8.0 cm and encircled many of the traversing pulmonary vessels.

They won't be able to surgically remove the mass, I thought. *This doesn't look good.* Trembling, I tried not to cry in the waiting room.

The pathologist concluded there was some form of cancer, but they didn't get enough cells to determine the type of malignancy. A week later, they performed a needle aspiration biopsy of the tumors, which involved poking a long needle directly into the lung.

Chris was in good spirits. Trying to lighten the mood, he played a trick on the anesthesiologist before the biopsy began. With the oxygen cannula in his nose, he spoke in a helium-type, high-pitched voice.

"I think there's something wrong with my oxygen."

The doctor looked startled for a few seconds and then started chuckling. He asked Chris to pull the same stunt on the radiologist. He obliged, and they all had a much-needed laugh.

On July 30, 2010, it became official. The pathology report confirmed malignancy—specifically, non-small cell carcinoma. His type was pulmonary adenocarcinoma—just a fancy term for lung cancer. My suspicion was confirmed: Chris wasn't considered a good candidate for surgery. Because of the tumor's location, they wouldn't be able to get all of it.

"The best treatment would be radiation and chemo to shrink the tumor and then reevaluate for surgery," said the doctor.

Neither of us cried when we got the official diagnosis. We already knew deep down the tumors were malignant because of his symptoms, so we were mentally prepared for the news.

The following morning, Chris went on a bike ride and made sure to ride a little farther than usual. He felt this would be a small victory over the cancer. He wasn't going to accept this diagnosis and simply give up on life.

> *"Have I not commanded you? Be strong and courageous! Do not tremble or be dismayed, for the* Lord *your God is with you wherever you go."*
>
> —Joshua 1:9

Chapter 4

A SIMPLE PRAYER

Chris prayed a simple prayer for God to place the right people in the right place at the right time and for something good to come from his experience with cancer. And so many times, He answered. The Lord knew who and what we needed before we did and was faithful to meet our needs, though not always in the way we expected.

We went out to eat a couple of nights after Chris was diagnosed. As we approached the restaurant, an obese man was smoking near the door. Unexpected anger and resentment toward that individual hit us hard. *He* deserved lung cancer, not Chris. That anger was short lived, however, because God quickly opened our minds, and we realized that no one deserves the disease. God allowed His own Son to suffer and die. We're His children too. We are no better than anyone else in God's eyes.

Instead of asking, *Why me?* my husband then asked himself, *Why not me?* That turning point helped us both understand there must be some reason Chris was chosen to have lung cancer. This was all part of God's plan for our lives. Maybe it was a test. Would we love or reject Him?

Chris decided to do something beyond just continuing to love God. He chose to turn his negative circumstance into something positive by writing a blog about his cancer journey and glorifying God in the process. This verse had special meaning to him:

> *I will not die but live, and will proclaim what the* Lord *has done.*
>
> —Psalm 118:17 NIV

While sharing what God was doing in his life, he educated people that never-smokers get lung cancer too. A "never-smoker" has never smoked. A "nonsmoker" may have smoked in the past but isn't currently doing so.

My sister-in-law LaDonna called me as soon as she heard about Chris's diagnosis. She was diagnosed in 2005 with non-Hodgkin's lymphoma and received treatment at MD Anderson Cancer Center in Houston. I believe her positive attitude through her treatment and recovery is a large part of the reason she's still alive today. Because of her, I knew what to expect and a few terms of medical jargon.

She gave me this piece of advice: "Keep a daily journal so you can tell the doctor how Chris's health status changes over time." So I tried to write down everything the medical team told us, what medications and treatments Chris was given, his vitals, weight, improvements, setbacks, and anything else I thought was worth keeping track of. My journal became a huge help during his treatment.

LaDonna suggested that we seek treatment at MD Anderson and gave me lots of other tips, including, "You can do a self-referral." That was a relief, since we didn't know where to begin seeking help.

She then recommended, "Don't have a PET scan done locally because MD Anderson will want to do its own scan. Insurance probably won't pay for two so close together. Don't surround yourself with negative people. If they start talking about how they knew someone with lung cancer who didn't live long, cut them short and let them know you need to focus on surviving."

We appreciated these last words of wisdom, but it was easier said than done.

"Chris is not a victim—he became a survivor the moment he was diagnosed," LaDonna said. "Each day he lives, he has survived cancer."

My brother Brett suggested that I not let my husband see me cry. "You need to be strong for him." That would be a tough order to fill; I cry easily.

That same evening, I was working in the yard when a neighbor stopped to chat during his walk. I mentioned Chris had been diagnosed with lung cancer.

"I received treatment at MD Anderson many years ago for cancer," Deke said. "While trying to decide where to go, a friend asked me, 'With the number one cancer center in the nation only four and a half hours away, why *wouldn't* you want to go there?' " It made sense to him.

It also made sense to us. That simple question confirmed in our minds that this was where we wanted to seek treatment. I searched on the MD Anderson website for lung cancer specialists. *No department is listed for lung cancer?* It frightened me. *Is it so bad they don't even bother treating it anymore?* After discovering that lungs fall under the Thoracic Head and Neck Department, I realized I needed to learn more medical terminology.

INFECTED WITH CANCER

A friend pointed out that Chris and I would say "we" went for treatment. That's because I attended every single appointment with him except one routine exam in our area. When we married, we became "one flesh." I was totally in this with him, and it would be a team effort to get him well.

There's also a saying, "When someone in your family gets cancer, it affects the entire family." That's so true. I was also "infected with cancer." Although I didn't go through the physical torture Chris endured, it was as mentally tough on me as it was on him. He was quick to point out he felt it was harder on the caregiver because they witness their loved one suffering. In addition to worrying about the present, they also have to consider a possible future without the person.

MESSAGES OF HOPE

One night as I tried to sleep, the last two lines of a song kept going through my head. Trying to figure out what it was, the words started surfacing in my memory. The tune was from the chorus of Bill and Gloria Gaither's "Because He Lives." I realized the "He" in the lyrics represented Christ, but if it were lowercase, "he" could also refer to my husband. A sense of peace overcame me as I fell asleep. *Chris is going to live.*

One Sunday after getting the initial CT scan results, the title of the church sermon was "Healed of a Lengthy Affliction." As Chris read the bulletin, he heard a voice out of nowhere say, *It will be a long, hard battle, but you will be healed.* The voice was so real to him, he choked back tears every time he attempted to tell someone during the next six years about that particular moment.

We met with the local pulmonologist on August 2 to go over all the findings, ask questions, and determine what to do next. Based on his chest scans, Chris was considered stage III. When we found that out, we launched a fact-gathering mission to conquer the beast in his chest. As an engineer, Chris analyzed data to fix a problem. That's how he approached meetings with doctors. It amazed me to watch his courage in the face of this life-threatening illness. *If he can be strong, then so can I.* But often, my shaky hands belied my calm demeanor as I took notes at appointments.

The next step was to have scans of the brain and entire body.

"There are good oncologists in the Dallas area, but I recommend you go to MD Anderson for lung cancer treatment," said the doctor.

"We've already decided that's where we want to go and did a self-referral online."

"My office personnel will speed up the process for you," he said. Before we left his office, he added, "You're in for a long, hard battle."

Hmmm. Chris had heard that already. Coincidence? We didn't think so.

CANCER ENCOURAGEMENT GROUP

That evening, I asked Chris to go with me to the Cancer Encouragement Group meeting at church. He was physically and emotionally drained.

"I don't want to hear a bunch of old people crying about dying of cancer," he said.

"Please go to one meeting to see if we can get anything out of it," I requested.

He complied, although he still didn't want to go. When we showed up, we found only a handful of people in attendance. We were the only newcomers that night, so they focused on how they could encourage us. The wall that we had built around our emotions tumbled down as soon as Chris told them his diagnosis. My husband and I were the only ones in tears and shaking with fear of facing an uncertain future. The others had beaten the disease. They shared their stories, which gave us encouragement, and they prayed fervently for us. When we left the meeting, we had hope.

> *The* L*ORD* *sustains all who fall and raises up all who are bowed down. . . . He will fulfill the desire of those who fear Him; He will also hear their cry and will save them.*
>
> —PSALM 145:14, 19

Chris voluntarily went to the next meeting with me. The group was much larger that night. People shared where they were in their journey, and one testimony stood out to us. Don was diagnosed in 2004 with stage IV throat cancer and was once told in the hospital, "You won't make it through the night." Don survived not only that night, but he's still alive and well as of this writing in 2018. This was more proof to us that God is the Great Physician and can heal even when the doctors have no hope.

We attended the meetings for the next six years, trying to become sources of inspiration and hope for others along the way to pay forward the help we received when life with a fatal diagnosis looked bleak.

MD ANDERSON TOUR

In mid-August, Chris was running a high fever and was down 20 pounds from his normal weight. I called the pulmonologist's office after hours to have him paged. I told the doctor on call that Chris had recurring pneumonia with lung cancer, so he called in a prescription at a nearby twenty-four-hour pharmacy. This kept us out of the emergency room. The antibiotics quickly helped the fever disappear, and by the time we arrived in Houston two weeks later, Chris was feeling better. He was ready to finally get things started.

Brett and LaDonna were also in Houston for her appointment at MD Anderson, and we stayed at the same hotel. They took us on a tour of the cancer center so it wouldn't be so intimidating, and we'd be able to find our way around more easily. My brother gave us each a special coin that represented the story "Footprints in the Sand." This was a tangible reminder that during the tough times ahead, it might seem like God had abandoned us. During those times, though, His love would actually be carrying us.

Footprints in the Sand

One night a man had a dream. He dreamed he was walking along the beach with the Lord. Across the sky flashed scenes from his life. For each scene, he noticed two sets of footprints in the sand, one belonging to him and the other to the Lord.

When the last scene of his life flashed before him, he looked back at the footprints in the sand. He noticed that many times along the path of his life, there was only one set of footprints. He also noticed that it happened at the very lowest and saddest times in his life.

This really bothered him, and he questioned the Lord about it.

"Lord, You said that once I decided to follow You, You'd walk with me all the way. But I have noticed that during the most troublesome times in my life, there is only one set of footprints. I don't understand why when I needed You most, You would leave me."

The Lord replied, "My son, My precious child, I love you and would never leave you. During the times of your trial and suffering, when you see only one set of footprints, it was then that I carried you."

—Author Unknown

In all their affliction He was afflicted, and the angel of His presence saved them; in His love and in His mercy He redeemed them, and He lifted them and carried them all the days of old.

—Isaiah 63:9

Chapter 5

DIAGNOSTICS AND MEETINGS WITH PHYSICIANS

On August 19, we met with Dr. Davis,* the thoracic oncologist who was assigned as Chris's main doctor at MD Anderson.

"Surgery might still be a possibility if the cancer hasn't spread. It would be the best option if the disease is confined to one area," he told us. "We'll be able to determine whether surgery or chemo and radiation will be the best treatment after surgeons review the PET and CT scans."

While there, Chris consented to do his part for cancer research. They performed a chest x-ray and drew nine vials of blood, five for the doctors and four for research. His heart rate was a healthy 57 beats per minute due to his bicycle riding.

We attended the new patient orientation and left with an abundance of information. One of the most useful items they gave us was a plastic page with twenty slots to hold business cards from the doctors, assistants, and office personnel we would be seeing. The pages were three-hole punched to put in a binder. I ended up buying more plastic pages because, over six years, I accumulated nearly a hundred business cards from medical professionals and referred to them often.

Heading home for the weekend, we had a sense of peace about the situation. Maybe we were just being naive, but we felt God was in control and that good would come out of this journey. For an unknown reason, this was all part of His plan, as Chris wrote in his blog post "Eye of the Storm."

> *I've tried to describe to friends the sense of calm that both DeLayne and I feel, but the only way I can think of is to say we're living in the eye of the storm. Where we are right now is calm.*
>
> *There's a great story in the Bible about Peter, my favorite disciple. The disciples have all gotten in a boat to sail to the other side of the sea. Jesus has stayed behind for the evening. In the middle of the night, the disciples see a figure walking on the water. At first, they believe it to be a spirit but then realize it's Jesus. Peter calls out to Him and tells Jesus that if it's really Him to say so, and he will come out to Him. The next thing Peter knows, he's out of the boat and walking on the water. Everything is fine until Peter takes his eyes off Jesus. Peter notices the wind and the clouds and starts to sink. He calls out to Jesus, and Jesus takes his hand and pulls Peter back to the surface.*
>
> *This story has really struck home with me the last few weeks. As long as I keep my focus on Jesus daily, I don't see the storm around me, and I sense the calmness of His love for me. But if I try to look too far ahead, all I see are the rolling, boiling storm clouds, and I feel scared with the uncertainty of it all.*

Chris also created a CaringBridge website to update family and friends about his medical status and to ask for prayer. It felt strange at first sharing medical details, but we felt we needed prayers more than privacy. In his online update, he kept his sense of humor.

"I was asked if I would allow them to use me as part of a study to determine why young, active, healthy, intelligent, handsome, funny, and humble people like me develop lung cancer. Yeah, I made some of that up, but you'll have to figure out which part."

GUARDIAN ANGEL

Back in Houston a week later, Chris woke me up at the hotel before the alarm clock sounded.

"Did you see him?" he asked.

"Who?"

"That man in the white robe."

At first, my husband thought it was a dream. He was in bed, looking at the door to the bedroom in our hotel. A man wearing a white robe with a belt tied at the waist was standing in the doorway. He slowly walked over to the side of the bed, bent over, and put his hand on Chris's chest. The sensation of being touched was so real it startled Chris awake. He concluded his guardian angel was telling him that he was watching over him in this battle. My husband felt he would be healed here on earth.

On the other hand, I immediately thought of my dad's experience. A couple of weeks before he passed away, Dad saw his mother walk across their living room floor, and he waved at her. She had passed away seventeen years earlier. I was afraid the man in our hotel room was a heavenly messenger telling Chris he would soon be escorting him to heaven. I never mentioned my fear.

ROLLER COASTER RIDE

We began the emotional roller coaster ride of cancer, which is filled with lots of ups, downs, and fast twists and turns. August 25 was a long day, starting at 6:20 a.m. with PET and CT scans. The brain MRI was the previous day. On the harrowing downward ride, we quickly gained speed when we received the results midafternoon. The radiologist didn't sugarcoat the findings.

"In just the last month," he said, "the disease progressed from the right lower lung to the middle lung and throughout the lung tissue. It's affecting the lymph nodes. New areas in the upper cavity near the esophagus and lower abdomen near the kidneys also look suspicious. There's also a three-millimeter suspicious spot on your brain. You're now considered early stage IV. Surgery isn't performed for stage IV patients."

Before we could begin to wrap our minds around this devastating news, he continued, "Ask your oncologist if chemo would be safe with a collapsed lung. Because lung cancer tends to come back time and time again, it requires chronic treatment. There's a possibility that microscopic disease elsewhere isn't showing up yet on the scans, and chemo could kill it. Chemo's your only option right now. I don't see a role for radiation at this moment, but it may be a possibility for the future." He felt Chris was strong enough to withstand the harsh forms of chemo.

Next, we saw the oncology surgeon. In two days, he planned to do another bronchoscopy down Chris's throat and a mediastinoscopy in which they'd make an incision below his throat and go in with a camera behind the heart to get biopsies of all the lymph nodes they could find. If they were cancerous, Chris would undergo chemo.

Instead of taking the shuttle back to our hotel a few blocks away, we walked. We didn't want to be around anyone. Holding hands, we dawdled in a solemn daze, totally silent. Reeling from the news, we were trying to absorb everything we'd been told. Hope was fading fast. I was seized with fear, my stomach in knots.

The disease is spreading aggressively. It's in his lymphatic system. It's in his brain now! Chemo is our only option. Chemo doesn't work very well on lung cancer. More suspicious areas are in his body. The brain—what do we do about the cancer in the brain? He went from stage III to stage IV in less than a month. Lord, help us!

SEEKING EDUCATION

We met with the anesthesiologist the next morning to go over Chris's medical history. Afterward, feeling overwhelmed, Chris went back to the hotel. He wanted to be alone with his thoughts. I decided to attend a class at MD Anderson to learn more about the disease.

As reality settled in, I was an emotional wreck, no longer numb from the initial shock of the previous day's news. But cancer wouldn't wait for me to gain control of my emotions. It would continue to threaten my husband's life at a rapid pace. I couldn't let fear paralyze me. Now was the time to take action to learn how to best treat it and enhance my husband's quality of life. I had a job to do as his caregiver, and I planned to give it my best shot. Being part of the team to save his life began with learning as much as I could about what we were facing.

Before the class started, I visited with two ladies who sat near me. Both were eager to share their stories.

The first woman had never smoked. After hearing that actress Dana Reeve's only symptoms of lung cancer were a cough and hoarseness, she went to an ear, nose, and throat doctor with the same complaints. When she asked if she had cancer, the doctor laughed and said, "It's only acid reflux. I've seen a lot of patients who suddenly think they have lung cancer since Dana Reeve's story was publicized." Still having the same symptoms months later, she went to a pulmonologist, and he diagnosed her stage IV lung cancer.

The other patient was a fifty-five-year-old woman who had smoked since age seventeen. She went to her doctor for help to quit smoking. Although she had no symptoms at all, he took an x-ray, which was cloudy but didn't indicate disease. A CT scan revealed stage IV lung cancer. I was amazed stage IV could have no symptoms, but I've heard similar stories many times since.

Next on my agenda was a class to learn how to give a massage to a cancer patient. The disease and its treatments can cause brittle bones, so it's important to be careful when applying pressure. We were taught to avoid pressing directly over a tumor. The instructor said to ask the oncologist if there are any restrictions for a massage, since the patient might have a condition that would preclude receiving one.

While listening to the instructor, I remembered the wonderful back rubs Chris had given me. *If he dies, I won't get those anymore.* I started crying. I was missing him already, and he was still alive. *How selfish to be worrying about my needs when Chris is in the battle for his life*, I realized, feeling guilty. I learned later that anticipatory grief is normal.

BIOPSY

Chris had the bronchoscopy and mediastinoscopy procedures on August 27.

"Only one lymph node biopsied behind the heart is positive for cancer. Surgery to remove the cancer is not an option," the surgeon confirmed. "There's no major blockage of the airway, and prognosis is good with targeted therapy."

Finally—a little bit of good news.

> *Blessed is a man who perseveres under trial; for once he has been approved, he will receive the crown of life which the Lord has promised to those who love Him.*
>
> —JAMES 1:12

Chapter 6

BATTLE PLAN

We headed back to MD Anderson filled with anxiety about what lay in store for us. What would be the battle plan? Could we tackle both the brain tumor and the lung cancer at the same time? If not, which was the more urgent one to control?

GAMMA KNIFE

Chris updated his CaringBridge page on August 31:

> *Today was a good day in the battle. Everything seemed to come up aces. First we met with the Neurological Radiation Oncologist. I'm definitely a candidate for the Gamma Knife procedure to treat the three-millimeter spot in my brain. He showed us the tumor is toward the middle of my brain. There's a slight risk of brain damage. He explained where the tumor is located there's minimal brain function and it's primarily "wiring." This part of the brain has built-in redundancy, so if any other cells get damaged, there are extras to compensate, and I wouldn't notice. That's most likely why I'm having no symptoms.*

In most cases where cancer has spread, brain tumors are treated first, and then standard chemo begins immediately after because chemo increases the risk of bleeding in the brain. If Chris were to start standard chemotherapy, he would have to be off chemo for two weeks before the Gamma Knife could be performed.

This procedure doesn't actually involve a knife. Instead, 192 pinpoint radiation beams with precision accuracy focus on the tumor from different directions like a sunbeam through a magnifying glass. With this stereotactic radiosurgery (SRS), neurologists can concentrate the radiation on a tumor. Nearby healthy tissue is protected from collateral damage, which is especially important in areas like the lungs and brain. The lack of an incision results in minimal discomfort and less risk of infection. Although SRS can only be used one time on a specific tumor, doctors can apply it to new tumors. If the tumors become too numerous or too large, whole-brain radiation is required—which can only be performed once.

After the doctor explained all this to us, he added the kicker: "The smallest brain tumor we've ever targeted was four millimeters. You may have to let the brain tumor grow."

"I'm not wild about that idea," Chris said.

The doctors presented his case to a review panel to see if they thought they could target a 3 mm tumor. They agreed to try.

TARCEVA

Earlier that month, a nurse from out of state (a friend of a friend) had sent information to us about lung cancer. She recommended a couple of useful websites, including cancergrace.org. This was established by Dr. Howard "Jack" West, a thoracic oncologist with a strong desire to help survivors worldwide. This information would become extremely helpful later.

She also shared a very important tip: "Mutations now play a very important part in treatment, so I would have the biopsy tested for the EGFR, KRAS, and ALK mutations right off. This helps determine if a new targeted therapy would work."

Having never heard of these three mutations, I looked them up. EGFR and ALK are more common in never-smokers, while KRAS is more common in smokers.

I had been researching the disease since Chris's diagnosis. He had started to research but then quit. It depressed him to see the poor success rate of available treatments and the survival statistics for stage IV lung cancer. He left this work up to me, and I told him things on a need-to-know basis.

The Thursday before Labor Day weekend, we met with Dr. Davis. Chris's resting heart rate was 95. He was obviously nervous.

I went in with a list of questions. Near the top was, "Will you test the biopsies for EGFR, KRAS, and ALK mutations?"

"We test for EGFR and KRAS here at MD Anderson, but we don't test for the ALK mutation because it's so rare. They only test for that in Denver. I doubt insurance would pay for the test. I think it costs about five thousand dollars," Dr. Davis said.

Since he was an oncologist at the number one cancer center in the nation, we trusted he had all the answers.

I asked if Chris could use the targeted therapy drug PF-02341066. The doctor wasn't familiar with it. I found out later that was Pfizer's code name for crizotinib, which was in clinical trials for ALK mutations.

After asking a few more questions, I bravely asked the one I was avoiding, knowing already that only God had the answer. "What is his prognosis?"

"I don't like to predict a timeline, but if we don't get things under control, things will start going bad in about six months."

I noticed he said "will" and not "could," and I panicked. My heart pounded so violently I thought it would burst through my chest. We were already four months past the time Chris's symptoms first appeared and one month past his diagnosis. I didn't have the courage to ask if Dr. Davis meant six months from when the symptoms began, six months from the date of diagnosis, or six months from that day.

My mind darted to the future. *Chad graduates from college in December. Will Chris live long enough to see him graduate?* I couldn't bear to think he might miss Shane's graduation or our sons' weddings. *He might never hear his grandchildren call him "Grandpappy."*

I snapped back to the present in time to hear, "You have two treatment options available at this point: standard chemotherapy or targeted therapy." The oncologist didn't want to wait two weeks for the Gamma Knife procedure before beginning to treat the lung cancer.

"Time is of the essence," he said. "Because the tumor has progressed since the last CT scan a month ago, we need to get started with the best therapy we have for this type of cancer. I want you to start today, if possible. Even though we don't have the results yet of the EGFR typing, as a young, healthy never-smoker, you fit the paradigm for having the type of cancer that will respond well to a targeted therapy drug called Tarceva. It targets the cancer cells but not the healthy cells and has few side effects. It's a once-a-day pill that you will take for three weeks. Then you'll come back for another CT scan to see if it's working on the tumor. If it's *not* working, we will either change treatments or add treatments. If it *is* working, you'll continue taking the Tarceva for at least six months. Because Tarceva isn't standard chemo, you can still do the Gamma Knife treatment for the brain tumor."

The oncologist encouraged Chris to ride his bike as much as he felt like. It would keep his heart and lung muscles strong, help him fight the cancer, and help him withstand the treatments better. Being out in the fresh air and sunshine would also keep up his spirits.

Excited, we left the consultation with a battle plan. We prayed the right person at the insurance company would approve the Tarceva in the next eighteen hours so Chris could get it and we could head home for the holiday weekend. But the plan came to an abrupt halt when we received a call at the hotel that afternoon. Our insurance was denying the specialty drug prescription for Tarceva because we didn't have the biopsy results confirming the EGFR mutation.

INSURANCE BATTLE

Dr. Davis faxed an appeal, and Chris called ABC Pharmacy* the next morning to confirm they received it. (ABC is the company that contracts with our insurance company to oversee pharmaceutical requests.) The man he spoke with said they hadn't received the paperwork and that it would be faster to have the MD Anderson (MDA) pharmacy call them. Chris called MDA's pharmacy and requested they call ABC.

Ninety minutes later, he called ABC again to see if they had the needed information. The woman who answered told him a phone call was not the acceptable method and that the information must be faxed.

Can't they agree on the procedure? I thought.

Chris called the MDA pharmacy again to pass along the new request. Then he called the oncologist's office to see if they had been able to get through to someone at ABC. No one answered the phone, so he left a voice message.

We were extremely frustrated that we couldn't get a straight answer. I couldn't just sit there and see Chris so disheartened. I felt I needed to do something to speed up the process, so I went to Dr. Davis's office to try to meet with someone face-to-face. The longer I sat in the waiting room, the more upset I became with the whole situation. *I'm trying to save my husband's life, but the insurance company and ABC won't cooperate.*

The oncologist and the physician's assistant weren't in the clinic that day. The nurse came out to speak with me. Agitated, I started crying as I explained the situation to her, and she called the doctor to fax another urgent appeal.

Early that afternoon, we learned the second appeal had been faxed, but it could take up to seventy-two business hours to process. Since this was a holiday weekend and many employees had left work, it might be the following Thursday before we received an answer.

I called our local pharmacy to see if they could have the medication ready as soon as the insurance approved it. Because of Tarceva's expense, they couldn't do that, but they did have a partial bottle of twenty-two pills in stock for some unknown reason.

Later that afternoon, we learned the second urgent appeal was also denied. At 4:20 p.m. on Friday, ABC called to say they were trying to reach Texas Instruments for permission to override the policy. The company was in charge of the insurance plan, so maybe there was still a ray of hope.

While we were grabbing a bite to eat before heading back to McKinney, MDA contacted us. Tarceva's manufacturer might give us the pills for free, but we would have to fill out paperwork. We gobbled down our food as quickly as possible and drove back to the cancer center only to learn we didn't qualify for the free medication.

We headed home, discouraged. My head was spinning, and I wanted off the roller coaster.

SLINGIN' ROCKS

What started out as a bad holiday weekend took a turn on Saturday. Chris's co-workers from his time at Texas Instruments in Sherman, Texas, surprised him with a visit. They cheered him up, reminiscing about old times together. When we discussed the fiasco with the insurance denials, someone suggested Chris contact Darla, a former co-worker who was now in the upper ranks in human resources in Dallas. He didn't know if she would even remember him.

The next morning, we went to church. Our pastor, Chuck Swindoll, gave a message we were sure he wrote just for us. The topic was David and Goliath and how we need to respond to the giants in our lives. His assertion that "no giants are larger than our God" and "the battle is the Lord's!" gave us hope.

Chris went home, proclaimed himself commander in chief of his body, and declared war on the army of cancer cells. With God's help, he was ready to start slingin' rocks.

On Labor Day, Chris started calling in the troops. He emailed Darla asking for help to override the insurance denial. "If I don't get this targeted therapy," he explained, "I'll have to choose between treating a brain tumor or the lung cancer first."

Although it was a holiday, Darla responded. She forwarded his request to the chairperson of the Benefits Appeals Committee, asking her to review the case quickly.

The chairperson wasn't in the office on Tuesday, so Chris contacted Art, his former supervisor, who had moved up within the company. Art, in turn, contacted the chairperson's co-worker and explained the situation, asking her to approve the recommended treatment for his former co-worker/friend. She immediately approved it. By 9:15 that morning, Chris received a call from ABC to let him know the Tarceva had been approved for thirty days, pending the results of the EGFR test.

It helps to have friends in high places.

MD Anderson transferred the prescription to our local pharmacy, and by lunchtime, I had twenty-two of the thirty pills to deliver to my husband. He was finally able to launch a counterattack against the giant in his life.

This valuable lesson taught us we would have to be our own advocates. In this instance, we had more power than the doctor in overriding the system. We learned to not settle for "no" when "yes" was in Chris's best interest.

We never found out why the local pharmacy had a partial bottle in its possession. Tarceva is a specialty drug and isn't normally carried in stock. This remains one of God's little mysteries.

The previous four days subtly reminded us that no matter the circumstances, God continued to put the right people in the right place at the right time.

> *This is what the* Lord *says to you: "Do not be afraid or discouraged because of this vast army. For the battle is not yours, but God's."*
>
> —2 Chronicles 20:15 NIV

Chapter 7

TREATMENT BEGINS

Within four days of starting the oral chemo, Chris developed "Tarceva skin" (dry skin and a severe rash). He put on so many lotions and potions, he created an oil slick in the shower.

"If you get a rash, it means the Tarceva is working," Dr. Davis said.

With roughly one-third of Chris's right lung collapsed, his voice sometimes cracked and squeaked from lack of air.

"Coupled with a rash that looks like acne, it feels like puberty all over again," he told the physician's assistant. "I didn't particularly enjoy that the last time and hoped to avoid it in my fifties. My cough is worse, but I'm breathing easier and deeper than I have in weeks. It's probably psychosomatic, since I'm finally doing something to fight the cancer."

"Who cares? Go with it," she responded.

So we did. It restored our spirits to at least *think* he was beating the disease.

PUTTING AFFAIRS IN ORDER

Since Chris was diagnosed with a potentially fatal disease and was now facing cancer in the brain, we decided to update his will while he was of sound mind. Although this was a grim topic to consider, we knew it was necessary, especially since he faced brain radiation in three days and could have complications.

I hired an attorney, and we each drew up a new last will and testament, since I was pregnant when we drew up our previous wills and our nineteen-year-old son was still named as a "future child." The attorney also created a directive to physicians, a durable power of attorney, and a medical power of attorney with a separate HIPAA release—all of which I might eventually need as a caregiver.

CONSOLING A NEIGHBOR

While visiting a neighbor, I told her Chris had stage IV lung cancer. She started crying, assuming stage IV meant he was in the end stages of life.

I tried to console her. "Stage IV simply means it's no longer contained to the point of origin," I said. "He's on a targeted therapy that has shown success in patients. We have hope for his healing."

It felt odd to be *giving* comfort instead of *receiving* it.

NOODLE NUKING

We spent most of September 15 at MD Anderson prepping for what Chris called his "noodle nuking." We also stopped by the thoracic unit to check on the EGFR mutation test. The cancer center didn't have enough tissue from the biopsy, so they contacted our local hospital to see if there were any tissue samples left from the biopsy done in July. There were.

It didn't seem right to pray for a positive result for a cancer test, but if the EGFR mutation was confirmed, we would keep doing what we were doing. A negative result would mean going back to square one on the treatment plan.

On September 16, the neurology team prepared to tackle the 3 mm brain tumor. A halo would hold Chris's head perfectly still during the radiation treatment. They attached it with four bolts screwed into his skull—two at the top of his forehead and two at the base of his skull. Although they deadened the area first, Chris almost passed out. It was partly at the thought of what they were doing, but also because his scalp was extremely sensitive from the Tarceva.

After the frame was bolted in and Chris's vitals stabilized, I was allowed in the preparation room. I watched a doctor put a plastic bubble over his head and measure the distance to his scalp from various angles. Chris later described it as a $68,000 Erector set with a goldfish bowl over his head.

Once inside the machine, his head frame was attached securely to a helmet to keep his head from moving. The procedure went well, although I don't know how Chris kept from coughing. He must have been saying some heavy-duty prayers for God to intervene.

> *"Do not be afraid. Stand firm and you will see the deliverance the Lord will bring you today. The Lord will fight for you; you need only to be still."*
>
> —Exodus 14:13–14 NIV

The neurosurgeon asked him how he felt after the radiation. The practical-joker side of Chris wanted to jerk his head like he was having a seizure while saying, "I'm fine." But he realized the doctor might not think that was funny.

The doctor informed us, "The original brain tumor hasn't grown, and we didn't find any new tumors. The tumor won't die immediately from the radiation. It will die over the next month or so."

We drove home the following day. Our next appointment wasn't until October 12. We would be able to spend almost an entire month at home—or so we thought.

Five days later, Chris felt fatigued and lost his appetite. The Tarceva had messed up his taste buds. He started running a high fever. MD Anderson advised him to go to the nearest hospital in case he was having a reaction to the Gamma Knife or had picked up an infection in the hospital. A brain scan showed no swelling or bleeding in the brain, but x-rays and a chest CT scan showed his pneumonia was worse. The good news was the lung tumor showed necrosis—it was dying. That meant the Tarceva was working. The hospital admitted him overnight and started him on a heavy dose of intravenous antibiotics. They sent him home the next day with oral antibiotics.

On September 30, the EGFR pathology test came back negative. We were stunned—this was not the news we wanted or expected to hear. We began praying that since Chris was in the small percentage of people with lung cancer who never smoked, maybe he'd also be in the small percentage of people without the EGFR mutation for which Tarceva was still effective.

CHANGES

Cancer negatively affected Chris's life in many ways. Although he still worked full time, some days he ended up leaving early and working from home. Other days, he worked all day from home because he didn't feel well or lacked energy. We changed where we sat in church so he could leave quickly if he developed a coughing fit or intestinal issues. He couldn't sing because it made him cough. He needed to eat every couple of hours to try to keep weight on. He actually got tired of eating.

Some changes initially appeared to be negative but proved to be positive, as Chris related in his blog post "Changes."

The lung tumor has caused part of my lung to collapse. This makes it difficult to speak sometimes. Singing is all but out of the question. Not being able to sing may be a positive for those around me, but I'm finding it also has a positive effect on me. Since I can't sing, I'm now more closely reading the words to the hymns, and I'm realizing what a wonderful gift the old hymns are to the church. Don't tell your music ministers I said this, but try this sometime: Stop singing and read the words. Let them soak in.

Then there are changes that can only be seen as positive. Sunrises and sunsets no longer just mark the beginning and ending of each day. They are times to be thankful for another day and celebrate the glory of God's creation. I know that my prayers and talks with God are a bit more direct and urgent. My quiet times and Bible study times are deeper now. I love Jesus and appreciate what He has done for me more than ever. I love and value my sons more now than the day they were born. I love my wife more each day and thank God every day that she's here for me to lean on. I simply can't imagine going through this without her by my side.

CHASING A DREAM

Chad was scheduled to graduate in December with a degree in mechanical engineering. Although he had already received a job offer from the company where he had interned, we weren't surprised when he called Chris in October to say that a couple of semiprofessional cycling teams had shown an interest in him. He didn't ask his dad's opinion of what he should do, but Chris sensed he wanted to. Our son apparently couldn't get up the courage to make this career change after we had put him through four years of college.

We had mixed emotions about Chad walking away from a good engineering job.

Chris said, "I don't want Chad to spend the rest of his life wondering, *What if?* Because of cancer, I'll probably never realize my own dreams of enjoying life in retirement. With his passion for cycling and his dream of becoming a professional cyclist, I don't want him to pass up a once-in-a-lifetime opportunity. He's in his peak fitness and has no responsibilities to prevent him from traveling."

I agreed.

Chris called Chad the following morning and gave our blessing. "Go for it and chase your dream. I have no doubt you'll make it."

HELPING HANDS

People arrived unexpectedly to bring us snacks or meals to show they cared. They mowed our yard, got our mail, and took care of our trash bins so it looked like we were home when we were in Houston. Our friend Deb Tolle set up an online meal train where people could sign up to coordinate meals for us.

In his blog entry "Friends," Chris wrote about how grateful we were for the friends and family who looked out for us:

> *Some of our friends have a knack for showing up when they know we need a laugh or a hug. Others seem to know when we can use a phone call to check up on us or an email to encourage us.*

In many instances, this "knack" was true. But on more than one occasion, I secretly contacted a close friend, our sons, or another family member to let them know Chris was having a rough day and could use a pick-me-up phone call or visit. No matter whose idea it was to reach out to us, it always rejuvenated our spirits to know others cared.

Two are better than one, because they have a good return for their work: If one falls down, his friend can help him up. But pity the man who falls and has no one to help him up!

—Ecclesiastes 4:9–10 NIV

NEW TREATMENT PLAN

Chris had lost 21 pounds. His cough was worse, keeping us awake at night. I thought he was going to cough up a lung, and I worried he was straining his heart. He was uncomfortable sleeping in bed, so one night he attempted to sleep sitting up on the upstairs couch while I tried to sleep in our downstairs bedroom with the door closed. Even though I wore earplugs, his coughing still kept me awake. It brought back the memory of how Dad sounded the Christmas before I lost him.

At times, I feared Chris wouldn't beat the cancer. Those were usually on the days when my research of available treatments revealed statistics of their failure rates. I kept reminding myself, *God doesn't need statistics because He's in charge and is still in the miracle business.*

Chris needed a miracle.

On October 14, we received another blow. The PET scan for restaging showed that Tarceva did *nothing* for Chris other than give him a rash and pimply face. So much for the theory, "If he gets a rash, it means the Tarceva is working." The tumor in his lung was *not* dying. It had grown from 6 cm to 9 cm in the past month. No wonder his cough was worse.

The new plan was to start him on two standard chemotherapies, paclitaxel and carboplatin, which Dr. Davis said he could receive in our hometown. When I asked if Chris needed a port installed in his chest, he replied, "A port won't be necessary. They will administer the chemo directly into a vein. A port puts the patient at greater risk of infection."

I booked an appointment the following day for a consultation with an oncologist in the Dallas area.

ONCOLOGIST WITH AN EGO

Shortly before our appointment with the local oncologist, I looked online for patient reviews. I found a poor review from one patient, who said the doctor had an ego problem. He had tried to get a copy of his medical records so he could get a second opinion elsewhere, but she was offended and refused to release the records to him. Since this was the only bad review I found, I didn't mention it to Chris. I didn't want to influence his opinion of the doctor before he met her.

The doctor agreed to treat Chris but wanted to put a port in his chest to administer the chemo. She also recommended a third chemo along with the other two chemotherapies Dr. Davis had ordered.

"Our doctor at MD Anderson didn't mention adding a third chemo, and he didn't feel a port was necessary," I said.

She bristled. "When he is in *my* office, *I* am his doctor and will follow *our* office protocol." She said she would check with Dr. Davis to see why the third chemo wasn't recommended.

I bit my tongue, but it worried me that maybe the negative review was right about her ego problem. *Does she think she knows better than our oncologist at the number one cancer center in the nation?*

She contacted our Houston oncologist and got his approval, although it was a challenge to reach him. We scheduled appointments for the port to be put in at our local hospital on October 25, with chemo to start the following day.

We never made it to those appointments.

GAMMA KNIFE RESULTS

Chris started running a high fever again the next evening at bedtime, so I called the local pulmonologist's office. The doctor on call was paged. When I explained that my husband had recurring pneumonia with lung cancer, the doctor called in a prescription for an antibiotic. Chris's fever disappeared the following day.

Back at MD Anderson for his checkup on October 21, we viewed the MRI images with the neurosurgeon's assistant. The brain tumor was either the same size or potentially smaller than the images taken the day of the Gamma Knife.

"There aren't any new spots present, and the radiation will continue to work over time. Bottom line is, the procedure was successful," she said.

Because Chris was doing so well, she didn't see a need for him to stick around for his appointment the following morning with the neurosurgeon. Chris was feeling great and was able to walk up two flights of stairs at the hotel four times during the day. We normally would have jumped at the chance to go home early.

God's hand was firmly on us, however, leading us to stay in Houston and keep the Friday appointment with the neurosurgeon.

> *Though I walk in the midst of trouble, You will revive me; You will stretch forth Your hand against the wrath of my enemies, and Your right hand will save me.*
>
> —Psalm 138:7

Chapter 8

BACK TO SQUARE ONE AGAIN

That night, Chris wasn't feeling well at bedtime and was up most of the night coughing extremely hard again. He wanted to take acetaminophen on Friday morning.

"Please wait until after your doctor appointment to take it, because it could mask a fever," I said. This was advice my sister-in-law LaDonna gave me when he was first diagnosed.

He didn't feel feverish at the time, but he abided by my request.

We arrived early for our 8:30 a.m. appointment on Friday, October 22.

Curled in a fetal position in the waiting room, Chris shivered with chills and looked ashen. "I feel like a freight train ran over me," he said.

He looked like it too. After the nurse called Chris in to take his vital signs, she sent him back to the waiting room. His pulse rate was 120 beats per minute with a temperature of 101.2 degrees.

Just minutes later, the neurosurgeon came out. "The good news is, the Gamma Knife worked. The bad news is, you're going straight to the emergency room."

We realized the Lord had kept us from going home. If we had cancelled the Friday morning appointment, we would've either been in McKinney Thursday night or on the road Friday morning when he developed the high heart rate and fever. If I'd let Chris take acetaminophen, the doctor wouldn't have known he had a high fever and would've sent him home instead of to the emergency room. We also wouldn't have received the top care of our Houston team, and things could've taken a completely different course.

It could have turned fatal.

Dr. John Heymach was the thoracic oncologist working the hospital shift at MD Anderson that weekend. We'd never seen him before Saturday. He told Chris, "The scans indicate a lung tumor is blocking your airway, creating a pocket of gunk the antibiotics can't get to, causing your recurring pneumonia." This doctor did *not* want a port installed on Monday or chemo started on Tuesday per the local oncologist's current plan. He continued, "The worst thing would be to halfway treat the postobstructive pneumonia and start chemo. The chemo would damage your immune system and make it harder to fight the pneumonia. It would be a train wreck."

We would have to put off starting the chemo for at least another two weeks or until the pneumonia resolved.

"I don't want you to get a port implanted yet, because it could create an infection," Dr. Heymach said. "I want to schedule a bronchoscopy on Monday to force open your airway and possibly put in a stent to keep it open. If the tumor won't allow this, we'll consult with a pulmonologist and radiologist to determine if they should use proton therapy radiation or intensity-modulated radiation therapy to shrink the tumor fast to open up your airway."

A pulmonologist came in later that afternoon. "I'm not sure the CT scan shows pneumonia," he said, "but the tumor has progressed from nine centimeters to thirteen centimeters. We'll do a bronchoscopy on Monday. If it's cancer causing the fever, we need to start chemo without delay."

The doctors weren't on the same page with their diagnosis and course of action. I began to panic. *Now what do we do?*

DESPONDENT

Sunday, October 24, was one of my lowest afternoons up to that point. Our sons drove from Texas A&M University in College Station to spend part of the weekend with us. Chris didn't feel well and didn't want the boys to see him hooked up to IVs. He had difficulty eating his lunch because the IV was in the crook of his arm. One of the boys stepped up to cut Chris's food for him. That simple act of kindness sent him into tears.

"It isn't supposed to be like this for another forty years," Chris sobbed. He covered his face with the blanket so the boys wouldn't see him crying. It broke my heart to see him so despondent.

Our emotions frequently mirrored each other's. I also felt melancholy because our sons would drive back to college later that afternoon, and I'd miss them. Every time they left, I experienced the empty nest syndrome all over again.

Chad and I made eye contact. I started tearing up and dashed out of the hospital room without saying a word. I needed to compose myself, but walking the deadly silent hallways on a Sunday made me even more forlorn. A sense of indescribable anguish suddenly enveloped me. I hurried outside for some fresh air and sunshine, only to find cloudy skies as dreary as my mood. Seeing the MD Anderson Cancer Center sign usually gave me hope, but that day it churned my stomach. I couldn't stand the thought of Chris having to be here.

He shouldn't have lung cancer! I screamed silently.

I rushed into the nearest bathroom stall to bawl in private. In the middle of blowing my nose, my cell phone rang. It was Chad. The doctor was in Chris's room to talk about treatment plans. I raced from the second floor of the cancer center's main building to his room on the sixth floor of the hospital next door.

REAR-VIEW MIRRORS

"I spoke with Dr. Davis, and he's in agreement with the bronchoscopy planned for Monday," Dr. Heymach said. "It's not uncommon for the thoracic oncologists to think the problem is pneumonia and for the pulmonologists to think the problem is cancer. I want to get a tissue sample during the bronchoscopy to send off to Denver to have it tested for the ALK gene mutation. This is a very rare mutation in nonsmokers—only three to seven percent of lung cancer patients have this mutation."

That was the mutation I asked Dr. Davis about on September 2, and he told us it was so rare they didn't test for it at MD Anderson.

Then Dr. Heymach added, "An oral treatment [crizotinib] that works for this mutation is in clinical trials."

Chris and I prayed they could get a firm diagnosis to determine treatment.

Later, we researched the ALK mutation.

"That's what I have—I know it!" Chris said. "It's so rare, I know I have it because I'm in the minority on the odds of having this disease in the first place."

I went back to the hotel that evening and called Dr. Bruce Douthit, a family friend. We talked about my disappointment in the local oncologist and her unwillingness to follow Houston's protocol. He then gave me recommendations for emergency rooms and hospitals in our hometown area. "If it were my wife with lung cancer," he said, "I would want her at MD Anderson. I did an internship there, and it's a great place for treatment."

I had seen how hard it was for Chris's local doctors to reach Houston staff. I had witnessed how quickly the various doctors at the cancer center collaborated and agreed to change his treatment plan. The conversation with Bruce confirmed what I felt. We needed to have all of Chris's treatment done at MD Anderson.

I called Chris at the hospital, but before I told him about my conversation with our friend, he told me he wanted to have all his treatment done in Houston. We were thinking alike. I then told him what Bruce had said, which solidified in his mind we were making the right decision.

Monday was the day Chris was supposed to get the port placed in his chest for chemo. Instead, he was getting a bronchoscopy.

"We didn't find any tumors in the airway during the bronchoscopy, so we didn't do a biopsy. We all agreed beforehand to not poke holes in your airway to obtain cancer tissue," the surgeon told Chris after the procedure. "We've requested tissue from the previous biopsy at your local hospital to send to Denver for testing."

He continued, "We discovered you have only a two-millimeter opening for your airway. As Dr. Heymach suspected, the tumor is pressing on your airway and closing it off, so antibiotics can't get rid of the pneumonia. We've decided the best next course of action is to radiate the tumor to shrink it fast so the airway can open. Then you can get rid of the pneumonia, allowing you to receive chemo."

They scheduled an appointment at the Proton Therapy Center the following morning for consultation and simulation.

We realized later that all the previous bouts with pneumonia had occurred at home. By the time we got to Houston, Chris's fever would be gone due to treatment with antibiotics, so the doctors at MD Anderson didn't realize how much the tumor had obstructed his airway. Once he got sick before their eyes, they realized what they were dealing with and quickly pivoted on the treatment plan.

God obviously had a strategy—we just weren't clued in.

Chris wrote "Rear-View Mirrors" after the chain of events that led to the sudden, complete change in his road map. Here's a snippet:

> *Looking in my rear-view mirror, I can see that God knew well in advance the doctor who would be on duty, his capabilities, and his knowledge. Too often I forget my simple prayer that God put the right people in the right place at the right time. Once again, He has been faithful to supply that person.*
>
> *Thinking about the rear-view mirror in my truck, I remember it has a compass in it. Sometimes you have to look backward to build your faith that God knows the direction going forward.*

For we walk by faith, not by sight.

—2 Corinthians 5:7

Chapter 9

RADIATION TREATMENT

We met with the radiation oncologist on October 26. He scheduled Chris for intensity-modulated radiation therapy (IMRT) because proton therapy had too narrow a focus for the large tumor. IMRT shapes the radiation beams to closely fit the shape of the cancer. Radiation would occur daily Monday through Friday for three weeks—a total of fifteen sessions at a fairly high dose.

I stayed with Chris during the radiation simulation. He reclined on something like a bean bag that conformed to his body. They marked a target on his chest with crosshairs and tattooed a permanent small dot under each arm pit and on his chest so that when he returned for daily radiation, he could be aligned with the equipment in that exact position.

Seeing Chris on the radiation table, I fought to hold back my tears. My doctors had suspected on two earlier occasions that I might have cancer. (I didn't.) I felt I should be the one on that table—Chris didn't deserve to be there, especially with *lung* cancer. It broke my heart to see everything he was enduring. He was a trooper, though. Typical of Chris, he kept the situation lighthearted by joking with the radiation techs.

The next day, they applied additional artwork to his chest, drawing with a red marker what I presumed was an outline of the tumor. It looked like a five-year-old child had drawn a big bull's-eye on his chest. Almost three months to the day of his official diagnosis, we finally launched a successful counterattack as Chris completed his first radiation treatment.

We had the privilege of meeting Bill Haines and his wife, Diane, in the waiting room that same evening. Bill was diagnosed with lung cancer just a month before Chris. He had developed an earache the previous year that wouldn't go away. None of the tests in his head and neck area showed the cause. The doctor finally did a CT scan eight months later and found that a tumor pressing on a nerve caused the earache. He was diagnosed at stage IV.

We hit it off instantly, feeling like we'd known each other for years. We used each other for moral support throughout our treatment in Houston.

By October 31, Chris was losing his confidence in the doctors and medicine. So was I. We weren't seeing his health improve. The radiation was physically wiping him out. After merely taking a shower, he had to sit on the edge of the tub to catch his breath before he could get dressed. His cough still sounded horrible, and he napped a lot, propping himself up in a chair or on the end of a couch with pillows so he could sleep.

He didn't look good. His color was gray, and he felt like a skeleton when I wrapped my arms around him. His shoulders were bony, and the muscles on his arms and thighs seemingly no longer existed. He was wasting away before my eyes.

I knew he was self-conscious about the drastic changes in his body, so I made sure he knew I loved him no matter how he looked. He was still the same wonderful man on the inside.

Chris was trying to figure out what lesson God wanted him to learn from all this suffering. *Is someone watching me to see if I will turn away from my faith in God? Will my healing draw someone closer to the Lord?* Whatever the lesson was, we just prayed God would throw us a life preserver soon. We were both starting to drown.

Chris was still working full time from our hotel in Houston. Most of his work involved communicating with people around the world via the computer. He was miserable and exhausted but was still trying to provide for our family, staying up late to put in the hours he missed during the day due to appointments or having to rest.

When Chris napped, I went out on the balcony to read about radiation treatments and side effects. I had difficulty concentrating. *The way he looks and acts, he isn't going to make it through the radiation treatments. He's getting worse instead of better.* I would cry my eyes out and then sneak back in the room to freshen my makeup before Chris woke up. I didn't want him to see tears quenching my hope.

CAREGIVER COUNSELING

On November 2, I attended a meeting for caregivers. I was the only caregiver who showed up, and I received some valuable tips during one-on-one counseling.

- Ask for medications to increase his appetite and mood.
- Get him to eat high-calorie protein foods such as smoothies and peanut butter.
- Read books on nutrition and coping with cancer.
- Talk to his doctor about how he's feeling depressed. The doctor is a tool in the arsenal to fight the disease.
- If he needs to, have him see a psychiatrist. There's a period of adjustment to cancer. It takes a strong person to realize they need help and pursue it.

- If you let it, the disease will suck the life out of you. You don't have to let it consume you. Have fun. He's a person *with* cancer. It doesn't define who he is.
- Distract yourself or do something constructive that you enjoy: Work puzzles, draw, paint, do photography, listen to music, listen to inspirational books on tape, play computer games, etc.
- Find the meaning of cancer in your life.
- Engage in the world outside of cancer. Don't let it rule your world. It's a choice you make. Are you going to have cancer, or let cancer have you? Take back your life from the disease as much as you can.

Those were all words I needed to hear. I left ready to do whatever was needed to take back our lives and help my husband beat cancer. We had a choice about how we responded to the new challenges we faced. Instead of becoming victims to the disease, we chose to become "more than conquerors" (Romans 8:37 NIV).

PUTTING ON WEIGHT

Because Chris looked malnourished, the first item on our agenda was for him to put on weight. I requested an appointment with a nutritionist at MD Anderson.

"You need to consume 2,400 to 2,600 calories each day with 77 to 90 grams of protein. Food, at this point, is to be considered as 'medication' and is to be taken on a schedule every two hours," she told him.

Most people would love to be told to eat every two hours, but it was a chore for Chris.

By November 10, Chris had difficulty eating and complained it felt like food was getting stuck in his chest. He weighed 30 pounds below his normal weight.

While sitting in The Park at MD Anderson—a large indoor area with tables, chairs, and a snack bar where patients and employees could relax—Nurse Celine* from the Gamma Knife procedure saw us and came over.

She shook her finger at him, looking stern. "You need to gain weight, or they'll put in a feeding tube. You don't want that."

"It hurts to eat," Chris said. "The radiation burned my esophagus, and it's painful to even swallow water."

"Tell your doctor. They have medication for that."

Still new to this cancer world, we didn't know he could take medicine to numb the pain in his esophagus so he could eat. In this massive facility, what were the odds of running into a nurse from two months prior who still remembered him and told us what we needed to hear? We considered Celine to be another one of God's earthly angels in the right place at the right time.

Putting weight back on Chris wasn't as easy as I thought it would be, especially in these days of low-calorie food trends. I tried to follow the nutritionist's suggestions to pack as many calories as possible into his food.

For example, she suggested adding powdered skim milk to shakes. Chris got irritated when he saw me using it because he said it changed the taste. One morning while he was taking a shower, I added dry powdered milk to a bottle of whole milk and mixed it quickly. He never noticed. Sometimes I had to resort to fooling him.

Since Chris didn't like cottage cheese, I ran it through a blender and hid it in garlic mashed potatoes topped with extra sour cream, cheese, and bacon bits. He had no clue cottage cheese was in there. He thought it tasted different because of the garlic. I also successfully hid Ensure in a coconut pie.

He never caught on to my tricks, and I never admitted what I did in case I needed to help him put on weight in the future. He gained 10 pounds in less than two weeks. Unfortunately, because I ate a lot of what he ate, I also put on weight.

The nutritionist instructed me to count Chris's calories and protein intake daily. He didn't like my reminding him to eat every two hours or asking what he ate, so I put a chart on the refrigerator. He logged what he ate at what time. I read the nutrition labels of each ingredient consumed and calculated whether or not he was on target to meet his daily nutrition goal. He then adjusted his eating accordingly.

RADIATION FEVER

Chris ran a fever daily after starting radiation, and it was getting harder to control it with just acetaminophen. With his cough getting worse, he ended up in the emergency room again.

The doctor suggested it was pneumonia since the x-rays were unchanged from the last time. "But," she said, "the only ways to confirm pneumonia are via biopsy and autopsy. I don't want to do either."

Neither did we.

She gave Chris a prescription for 500 mg (milligrams) of Levaquin. I consulted my journal notes in the three-ring binder I carried with me to his medical visits.

"Can he get a prescription for 750 milligrams instead?" I asked. "That's the dosage prescribed in the past that helped him."

The doctor readily agreed to change the prescription. My detailed records were proving beneficial.

On November 16, Chris finished his fifteenth radiation treatment. He celebrated by ringing a bell three times to signify that cancer was now on the run.

THE PHONE CALL

The next day was his fifty-first birthday. About two hours after returning home from Houston, we received the call we were waiting for from Cheryl,* the physician's assistant.

"The biopsy results show you *do* have the ALK mutation," she said. "You still have to go through at least two rounds of standard chemo with two different chemotherapy agents and be restaged to see if the chemo is working. You'll only be eligible for the crizotinib clinical trial if there continues to be progression of disease, proving standard chemo didn't work."

Cheryl continued, "You have to wait at least two more weeks to start chemo. This will give you time to get your strength back after radiation and get over the pneumonia. We've already started the paperwork to get you accepted into the clinical trial, if necessary, so there won't be a delay."

Chris was elated. We cried tears of joy as we embraced. God had answered another prayer. No more guesswork. We knew exactly what we were fighting. Chris couldn't have received a better birthday gift. Having the ALK mutation put another tool in our tool box—potentially a sledge hammer.

Our insurance *did* pay to test for the ALK mutation. We learned from this experience to never let a doctor limit our treatment options based on cost and the assumption we can't or don't want to absorb the extra cost if insurance doesn't pay. Doctors don't know what each company will or won't pay for, and the doctor also doesn't know the patient's financial situation. A doctor should give the patient all available possibilities and let the patient's family decide if they want to pursue a costly but potentially lifesaving test or treatment.

As strange as it may seem, that night we prayed the standard chemo wouldn't work. We wanted Chris to get into the clinical trial, which had promising results.

And I was kicking myself for not insisting he be tested for the ALK mutation earlier.

MAKING A COMEBACK

Chris had been fever-free for three days and felt good enough to go to church on November 21. He was also able to sing.

Something most people take for granted was a monumental achievement for him.

He was able to walk around the neighborhood, vacuum downstairs, help me wash dishes, and fold laundry. That was quite an improvement from a week earlier when merely taking a shower and getting dressed exhausted him. His cough was greatly improved. He was making a comeback.

We had a great Thanksgiving. Both boys were home from college, and we celebrated the holiday with family. Chris found that xyloxylin, one of the medications prescribed to help numb esophageal pain, worked best if he took it forty-five minutes to an hour before a meal. Once it kicked in, he had about forty-five minutes to eat as much as he could. Sparks flew from his utensils during that time, and he warned everyone not to get their hands close to his plate.

BLACK FRIDAY

I normally decorated the house the day after Thanksgiving so I could enjoy the Christmas season as long as possible, but that year, Black Friday was a dark day for me. I had dreaded December for a couple of months. It would be my first Christmas since Dad had passed away, and I didn't know if we could be with Mom in Oklahoma for emotional support. I had never spent Christmas away from my parents.

Every year, my husband watched *It's a Wonderful Life* by himself. I don't enjoy watching the same movie over and over, and I also find that movie depressing. But I had intended to watch it with Chris that day until I read his blog post from earlier that morning about the film. It upset me. In his post, he asked, "Would it matter to anyone if I were not here? Have I made a difference to anyone?"

The mere thought of him not being here tore me up. I went into our bedroom, closed the door, crawled into bed, and cried myself to sleep. When I woke up, I could hear Chris watching the movie in the living room. The boys had gone for a bike ride, so I knew he was alone. I heard the little girl in the movie plodding "Hark! The Herald Angels Sing" over and over on the piano, and it made me start crying again. I hated that he was watching the movie by himself, but I just couldn't handle it.

Chris realized he hadn't seen me for a while and came to see what I was doing. He found me bawling. He climbed onto our bed and snuggled next to me to comfort me. I confided I had been trying to be brave for him, but inside I was terrified he might not survive. The thought of life without him was more than I could handle. To know he questioned whether or not he made a difference to anyone upset me. He had made a big difference in my life.

STRONG SUPPORT SYSTEM

Seeing Chris so weak during radiation was scary. Formerly robust and full of vitality, he was skin and bones, sleeping a lot, and looking like "death warmed over." I struggled to keep a strong front, holding a tsunami of emotions in. Occasionally, billowy waves crashed over me, destroying my façade.

Many mornings I'd have a smile on my face as I kissed Chris good-bye before I went to work. But as soon as I got in my car, tears started flowing, and I cried all the way to the office. My client and his wife, Jay and Lou Ann, were so compassionate. Having worked with them for eleven years in their home-based office, we'd become close friends. Seeing me walk in the door with a shiny red nose and bloodshot eyes, they knew I was having a rough morning and let me cry on their shoulders while they comforted me.

The material I had read on combating cancer stressed the importance of having a strong support system. Our system at home was invaluable, with people providing meals and professional massages, sending emails and notes of encouragement, calling and visiting, sending CDs of church services we missed, and praying for us. Friends and family got us through tough times and played a vital role in Chris's recovery. Their food nourished our bodies, but their kindness touched our hearts and revitalized our spirits.

We were amazed by people we'd never met who reached out to us. One special prayer warrior was Amy Smith, a friend of Janet Johnson, whom I've been friends with since we were both in kindergarten. Janet asked Amy to pray for us, and she did. She left encouraging notes on Chris's blog and occasionally mailed cards, saying she was praying for us. A year after Chris passed, I spent a weekend with Janet and Amy, and we had such a sweet time together. What a blessing to finally meet the woman who had faithfully prayed for my husband and me. His death had left such a hole in her heart that her own husband asked her, "How do you know this guy?"

"I don't know him—but I *do* know him," she answered, weeping.

Such was the impact Chris's blog had on her and her own spiritual walk. The power of her heartfelt prayers and notes of encouragement from this complete stranger touched us just as deeply.

We were worried about not having a support system in Houston. But thanks to Chad's college friend Devin Carroll, who had moved to Houston with his bride, Stephanie, a support system developed. Stephanie brought us a home-cooked meal at the hotel. Then her Bible study group adopted us. Devin's mother, Patty, whom we had never met, drove forty-five minutes to bring us food she'd prepared herself. She even brought me a gift basket of bath items to pamper myself.

We were grateful we didn't have to go to a restaurant for every meal. Leaving the hotel was physically exhausting for

Chris during radiation, and deciding what to order was more than he could mentally handle when he didn't feel well.

It was hard for us to learn to accept help from others, but through talking with those who were blessing us, we learned that we were, in turn, allowing God to bless them. What a disservice it would have been to deny them an opportunity to experience the joy of helping someone in need.

> *In everything I showed you that by working hard in this manner you must help the weak and remember the words of the Lord Jesus, that He Himself said, "It is more blessed to give than to receive."*
>
> —Acts 20:35

Chapter 10

CONFESSION

I used to open my Bible only on Sundays. I tried reading through the Bible many times over the years but lost interest because I was reading it as merely a historical book instead of the living Word of God.

We were driving to Houston once again, a captive audience listening to sermons on our favorite Christian radio station.

Robert Jeffress preached first. "It's important to read your Bible every day, preferably first thing in the morning before your day starts."

Chuck Swindoll was next. "I suggest reading your Bible first thing in the morning before starting the day," he said.

Then came David Jeremiah's sermon. "The ideal time to read the Bible is first thing in the morning before your day starts."

Finally, Charles Stanley came on. I'll give you one guess what the sermon was about.

"Okay, God, I got the message," I shouted. His voice may not have been audible, but His message came through loud and clear. I needed to deepen my knowledge and strengthen my spiritual walk to make it through the tough times ahead. I made a commitment to start reading the Bible every day. I didn't allow myself to get on the computer until I'd read my Bible. It quickly became a habit.

There's rarely been a morning since when I haven't jumped out of bed, snuggled up in my chair in the living room with my *Life Application Bible* and pencil, and treasured spending time with God's Word. What made the time more special was seeing Chris sitting in his chair at the kitchen table doing the same thing. It started our day off right.

My husband had been faithful to read his Bible daily for as long as I can remember. It's sad to think it took a cancer diagnosis to get me to follow his example. *Is that the reason God let Chris have cancer?*

The book of Job reminded me that Christians were never promised an easy life. Even if my husband didn't survive, God was in control, and it would be part of His plan. He would take care of me. I learned when in times of tribulation, don't close your Bible—open it.

God's precious promises in the book of Psalms were a great comfort to me during our crisis. I personalized them like Chris did. Whenever the Scriptures referred to evil, the enemy, the wicked, etc., I substituted the word "cancer." When he developed new medical issues and it was hard to focus on the Bible, I defaulted to Psalms to remind me there's hope.

However, doubts still slithered into my thoughts, gnawing at my belief that God would heal Chris, and it became challenging to concentrate on any Scripture at all. In the front and back covers of my Bible, I listed everything I was thankful to the Lord for providing over the years: family and friends, jobs, a roof over our heads, reliable vehicles, insurance, good medical teams, successful treatments, more time with Chris, church leadership and Christian mentors, our military, and our freedom—just to name a few. In dark hours filled with fear, I would read over the list and make a conscious effort to thank the Lord for all He had provided. It's amazing the mental transformation that takes place when your heart exudes gratitude.

> *I sought the* Lord, *and He answered me, and delivered me from all my fears.*
>
> —Psalm 34:4

Chapter 11

STANDARD CHEMOTHERAPY

Chris's appointment to start chemotherapy on December 2 was cancelled. In reviewing the radiation reports, Dr. Davis saw that between 98–99 percent of the lung tumor was in the field of radiation. To qualify for the clinical trial, we had to prove standard chemo wasn't working. Since radiation can continue working for up to six weeks after the last treatment, we wouldn't be able to determine if the tumor was shrinking from chemo or from radiation. If we couldn't use the lung tumor as an indicator, then another site would have to be chosen.

When Chris was first staged, they found lymph nodes in his chest and abdomen that were suspicious. He underwent another scan of the brain, chest, and abdomen. If the lymph nodes had grown worse, they could be used for the sites to judge chemo. If they were the same or no longer suspicious, then we would be looking at delaying chemo until after the first of the year.

The doctor told us Chris was his first and only ALK-positive patient. One good thing came out of his diagnosis—Dr. Davis started reviewing other patient records to see if he needed to send in their biopsies for testing for the ALK mutation.

"The first lab rat does eventually get his cheese, right?" Chris asked.

STANDING IN HONOR OF CHRIS

Two days later, Stephanie Carroll sent an email to me. "The sermon this morning was on healing. Devin and I stood in Chris's honor at the end of the service, and our friends laid hands on us, praying for him (and you). We believe God can heal Chris, and we are asking that He will."

> *This is what the* Lord, *the God of your father David says: "I have heard your prayer and seen your tears; I will heal you."*
>
> —2 Kings 20:5 NIV

STANDARD CHEMO STARTED

The doctor's office called on December 7 with the CT scan results. All the spots in the previous CT scan were stable, but two more spots less than 1 mm in size had appeared in Chris's chest. The doctor recommended he begin standard chemo, a combination of paclitaxel and carboplatin, since we had new tumors to use as a baseline for the chemo's effectiveness. We scheduled the first treatment for December 16, with the assurance that with the proper medications Chris would feel well enough to attend Chad's college graduation the following day.

During the chemo, we watched episodes of an old favorite TV sitcom and listened to Christmas carolers who graced us with their presence. It was a pleasant day, despite the fact Chris's body was being poisoned with chemicals.

Three days after chemo, he felt good enough to ride two laps around the neighborhood on his bike, which was great for both his body and mind.

THE THREE AMIGOS

The most noticeable side effect from the chemo appeared two days after Christmas, when Chris could pull out clumps of hair with little effort. He had determined early on that *he*—not the cancer—would be the one to decide when to go bald. I was afraid it would depress him to lose his hair, but he took it in stride. Chris and our boys broke out the electric clippers and engaged in one of the greatest father-son bonding activities of all time—head shaving. They took turns shaving each other's heads in different goofy hairstyles while I photographed the craziness. We laughed for a solid hour.

What could have been a depressing event turned out to be one of my fondest memories of the journey. We knew we had great kids, but they went above and beyond our expectations. What an act of love to shave their heads in support of their father. They also confirmed that they inherited their dad's off-center sense of humor.

If laughter is the best medicine, we gave the cancer a heavy dose that afternoon.

> *A joyful heart is good medicine, but a broken spirit dries up the bones.*
>
> —Proverbs 17:22

THE PROCESS

We saw Dr. Davis the first week of January 2011 before Chris's second round of chemo.

"We're getting the paperwork ready for the crizotinib trial in case the chemo isn't working," he said. We wanted to get in the phase II study. He explained the different phases of the studies:

- Phase I: The drug is tried for the first time on humans to see the side effects and to find the maximum tolerated dose that is effective.

- Phase II: Tests to see how well the drug works. You're usually guaranteed the drug.
- Phase III: Compares the trial drug to standard chemo. The patients are randomly selected for the experimental treatment or for chemo.

Chris wrote a blog entry titled "The Process," where he compared the process involved with cancer treatment to a spiritual process:

While I was recovering from the radiation treatments and preparing to begin chemotherapy, I completed my study of the Psalms. During this time, I became even more convinced I'll be healed from cancer. This conviction led me to ask the following question of God: If You're going to heal me, why put me through radiation, chemo, and all of these tests and treatments? Why not just heal me now?

Then one morning when I woke up, the first thing to come to mind was Lazarus. That thought seemed out of place with what I'd been reading, so I ignored it and pushed it out of my mind. I'll admit I'm not the sharpest tack in the box sometimes, but when it happened two more mornings, I finally took the hint and opened my Bible to the story of Lazarus in John 11 and 12.

The first thing I noticed is that Jesus knew the sickness wouldn't end in death but for the glory of God, and so the Son of God would be glorified. Also, even though Jesus loved Lazarus, He waited to go to him.

I, too, will wait so the Son of God will be glorified in my healing. I'll admit I don't like waiting. I want this process to move faster than it is, but at each phase of my treatment, we learn something new that we wouldn't have learned if we were moving faster.

The second thing I noticed is Lazarus' sisters asked a variation of my question to Jesus. "If you had come sooner, you could have healed him." Jesus tries to explain to them about the resurrection and life. When they and the crowds with them continue to weep, He sees their doubt and is deeply troubled.

It strikes me that my question shows I also have some doubt about God's plan and the process He's putting me through. Sometimes doubt enters my thoughts, but I still maintain the faith in my heart. The one thing I don't want to do is grieve Jesus with my doubt.

The final thing I noticed is that the chief priest started making plans to kill Lazarus. Why? Because he had become a witness for Jesus. Large crowds were gathering to see him. This part makes me smile a little. I like to imagine Lazarus being at dinner or out on the street, and a large crowd gathers to look at him. Finally, someone musters the courage to ask him, "Hey, aren't you the Lazarus that died?" And he answers, "Yes, I am, and let me tell you what Jesus did for me."

This makes me look forward to the day that someone comes up to me and says, "Hey, aren't you the Chris Haga who had lung cancer?" And I can answer, "Yes, I am, and let me tell you what Jesus did for me."

Most of all, through all of this, I'm learning that God has a plan for the rest of my life. He only reveals to me what I need to know for each day. It's become evident to me that part of the plan includes a process of refinement for me. The process isn't pleasant and can be real uncomfortable at times. I want it to move faster than it is. I know when it's completed that I'll be a better witness for Jesus.

I awoke one morning with these words in my head: To rush the process would be to ruin the process.

I will wait, watch, listen, and pray to be ready when the process is complete in His timing.

Even though we had experienced what seemed like setback after setback, we were slowly coming to realize that this was all part of God's perfect plan to bring Him glory. Just think, if Jesus had saved Lazarus before he died, the testimony wouldn't have been as amazing. Sometimes we have to experience a low point in our lives to make our witness for Christ more powerful.

I don't like to give up control, so it was challenging for me to not rush the process. Tired of waiting to see what He was up to, I prayed for no more setbacks so Chris could start the study right away. Apparently, God had other ideas.

ANOTHER CHEMO—ALIMTA

On February 3, plans changed again. The brain MRI showed no active cancer. The PET scan revealed the lung tumor mass was no longer active and had shrunk from 9 cm to 3.6 cm. The x-ray of his chest showed improved air movement in the right lung. His lungs had more fluid, which is normal during recovery from radiation. The fluid was settling to the bottom of the lung, allowing easier breathing. His blood tests were mostly normal. The suspicious lymph nodes in the previous scan had decreased activity. But a new suspicious spot had appeared in his liver.

I remembered Dr. Davis told us if Chris had no drastic improvement from the chemo, he would be a candidate for the clinical trial. Since he did have a drastic improvement, maybe God threw in a suspicious liver spot to qualify him for the study. The spot was apparently so small that Cheryl, the physician's assistant, couldn't see it on her computer.

Dr. Davis was ill that day, so Dr. Murray* filled in for him.

"With the new spot appearing during chemo, the mixed response will help you qualify for the clinical trial," Dr. Murray said. "To qualify for the phase II trial, you need to have been on two different chemo *regimens*—not just two different chemo *drugs*. Paclitaxel and carboplatin combined only count as one regimen. The chemo will be changed to Alimta to meet the criteria." He paused. "I don't know if crizotinib will work in the brain, but Alimta works across the blood-brain barrier, so you're in a good spot with this treatment."

Cheryl chimed in. "We don't expect nausea or vomiting. This is considered to be a maintenance drug that can be stayed on for years because the blood counts don't go down with it. Fatigue is the most common side effect experienced."

They rescheduled the new chemo for later that day. Alimta was normally given every three weeks. Cheryl didn't expect Chris to have any problems on it, but because chemo has cumulative effects, she suggested a four-week cycle to allow his blood counts time to recover. Pfizer, the drug manufacturer of crizotinib, wanted to do its own gene analysis on Chris's biopsy tissue, and that would take four weeks. A four-week cycle would also give Pfizer time to obtain the tissue from our local hospital and analyze it.

Although this was one more delay and required more standard chemo, I was grateful for God sending Dr. Murray to guide us on the correct path needed to guarantee a quicker acceptance into the clinical trial.

PROVIDING THE WAY

When we met Anne, the clinical trial nurse, she told us, "If you weren't seeking treatment at MD Anderson or another major cancer center that has this clinical study, you wouldn't be able to get crizotinib. This drug is showing to be highly effective in reducing and controlling disease for people with the ALK gene mutation."

I responded, "I read a report that showed one patient has become cancer-free on crizotinib. Chris will be number two. Mark my words." That may have been a bold statement, but I believed God would grant that miracle.

"Mr. Haga, you were highly selected to participate in the trial," Anne said. "We'll do whatever it takes to get you in the phase II trial instead of phase III so you'll be guaranteed to get the drug. Only two hundred people nationwide will be selected to participate. MD Anderson is allowed twenty participants. You'll be our fifth one."

Chris would need to have all the scans again the following month for restaging. We were concerned our insurance wouldn't pay for the same tests so soon.

"That's not a problem. The study will pay for the testing as well as for the cost of the experimental drug," she said. "You have nothing to worry about. I'll make sure you're taken care of."

And she did.

Next, we met with the neurosurgeon for a follow-up on the Gamma Knife. The tiny spot in his brain was smaller than before and was probably just scar tissue that would remain. Otherwise, the brain MRI looked perfect.

All in all, we felt God was being so good to us. He knew our every need and provided for us even when we didn't know what to ask for.

NEUTROPENIA

Chris developed a chest cold, and I caught it. My cold got better after a week, but his got worse. He coughed so hard he hurt his back a couple of times. We expected his immune system to be at its lowest on days seven through ten of his chemo cycle. He was on day nine. According to tests done in Houston the prior week, we knew he had more fluid in his lungs. We were afraid he would develop pneumonia. He had been running a fever for four days, and doctor's orders were to get to an emergency room if his fever reached 101 degrees because it could turn into a life-threatening situation. When he ran a 100.5-degree fever on February 11, we decided to head it off at the pass and went to the ER.

Although several other couples were in the waiting room, the ER personnel immediately whisked Chris into an isolation ward. Apparently, lung cancer patients with a cough and high fever during flu season get high priority in triage. Although they said it was possible he had pneumonia, he was diagnosed with neutropenia. His absolute neutrophil count was dangerously low, which meant his immune system was almost nonexistent.

We were shocked. Cheryl at MD Anderson had indicated he wouldn't become neutropenic on Alimta. "It's a mild chemo, as far as chemo goes," she had said. My husband was that rare patient where Alimta affected his immune system.

Shortly after midnight, an oncologist came in to see him.

"Chris didn't actually reach a 101-degree fever before we came," I said. "Did we jump the gun?"

She assured me we made the right decision. "I tell my patients to come in if their fever reaches 100.5 degrees." And she was bluntly honest about the severity of his condition. "It's possible for a neutropenic patient to look and feel well, get an infection the body can't fight, and then suddenly take a turn for the worse and die. If you had waited until he looked or felt really bad, it could have been too late."

I wore a hospital mask the entire time I was at the hospital.

"Are you sick?" the doctor asked me.

"I'm getting over a cold."

"Don't get near your husband or touch him. I would prefer that you leave."

Although I had planned to spend the night with him, I left per her instruction. His health was her main concern. It was also mine.

On Sunday, one of the nurses saw Chris reading his Bible. She mentioned she had watched a church service on television regarding praying for healing.

"Do you have faith you'll be healed?" she asked him.

"Yes."

She walked over to his bedside and, with his permission, placed her hands on his chest. She prayed for his complete healing. He was deeply touched. He never had a nurse do that before and doubted they taught that in nursing school.

Since I wasn't allowed at the hospital, I did some deep cleaning to rid our home of cold germs. Cynthia, a neighbor I barely knew, came over to our house to help me disinfect door knobs and anything else Chris might touch. She had recently lost her son to cancer and knew, from experience, how exhausted I would be and how important a germ-free environment was.

We felt so blessed to know such caring people.

VALENTINE'S DAY IN THE HOSPITAL

Chris was still in the hospital on Valentine's Day. Although I was over my cold, I still wore a mask to prevent breathing any germs on him. His blood counts had gone from too low to too high.

I gave him a heart-shaped box of chocolates decorated with the words "Faith, Hope, Love." Those words described exactly what we had. I wrote a letter to Chris and put it in his card:

> *All the things that have happened in our family in the last year are not things that I'd wish for anyone. But yet I feel lucky because of what has happened. It's made me appreciate you more, and it has made me thankful for every moment I get to spend with you—whether it's cuddling with you or just sitting in a waiting room or hospital room together, not speaking a word.*

I always felt I wasn't a strong person emotionally and could never handle situations such as the deaths of our dogs and my father—all within seven months. Then add a stage IV lung cancer diagnosis for the love of my life. It has made me realize that I am strong—but only with the Lord's arms wrapped around me to hold me up when my knees just want to buckle. I couldn't have gotten through this last year without you and without the Lord by my side.

I often wonder if I'm the one the Lord is trying to reach through your ordeal. All I know is, I am now in prayer a lot more often and enjoy being in the Word every morning. Thank you for showing me the Way by your example. Thank you for being a wonderful husband and father and a great role model for our boys. I am truly blessed to call you "mine."

If there were nothing else but our love for each other, I would still have all I need. Wherever life leads us, just being with you is all I want.

I have faith that God will heal your earthly body. I have hope that we will grow old together. And I will love you for my entire lifetime.

I love you, and I thank God for you.

And now these three remain: faith, hope, and love. But the greatest of these is love.

—1 Corinthians 13:13 NIV

Chapter 12

FIRST CLINICAL TRIAL

At MD Anderson on March 1, 2011, technicians scanned Chris from the top of his head to practically the tip of his toes, including a baseline eye exam.

Two days later, the test results were all good, giving us a surge of hope. We had a lot to be thankful for. For the first time, the scans didn't find any new cancer sites. Previously active areas showed either decreased activity or none at all. The spot in his liver discovered the previous month was no longer active. His blood tests were mostly normal.

This chemo worked—but that would prevent him from qualifying for the clinical trial. He could only get in if the disease progressed on standard chemo.

The low blood count caused by Alimta was rare for that chemo, but it was another blessing in disguise. It worked to fight the cancer, so we could use it again, if necessary. And the "adverse reaction" of neutropenia helped meet the requirements for the clinical trial. The final piece to God's puzzle was now in place. Things were looking up, and so were we. Only God could have orchestrated such an intricate plan.

Pfizer's biopsy results confirmed Chris tested positive for the ALK mutation. He was accepted into the study for the ALK inhibitor drug crizotinib and started the pills that same day. This targeted therapy drug inhibits the growth of the malignant cells specific to his ALK gene mutation. He was officially the sixth patient in the MD Anderson study. In the prior month, more than fifteen patients were identified with the ALK mutation. The study was limited to twenty patients and was now closed to new participants. If Anne hadn't started the paperwork the previous month, Chris wouldn't have been accepted into the study.

As we were going over the paperwork and instructions for the clinical trial, she advised us to avoid conceiving a baby while Chris was on the medication.

"Since I've had a hysterectomy," I said, "that's not a concern."

She then turned to my husband. "Don't get anyone else pregnant."

Chris chuckled. "If I got another woman pregnant, I wouldn't have to worry about cancer killing me. My wife would kill me first."

MORE THAN WE COULD HANDLE

Now that life was getting back on track again, we could take a deep breath and relax a bit while reflecting on all we had been through and how we had managed to survive. There's a popular saying, "God never gives you more than you can handle." We were finding this was far from the truth.

Here's an excerpt from what Chris wrote in "More Than I Can Handle."

> *If God doesn't give me more than I can handle, then what has been the role of my friends and family who have hoisted us on their shoulders while on their knees in prayer? If I could handle this on my own, there wouldn't be any need for these numerous people who have rallied around us to offer us support and food at home and in Houston. No, I can't handle cancer by myself.*

If God doesn't give me more than I can handle, then what role is there for Jesus? If I were able to fix this on my own, exactly when would I learn to depend on Him? Jesus, Himself, said, "Come to Me, all who are weary and heavy-laden, and I will give you rest" (Matthew 11:28). I'm so thankful for that invitation. There are days that cancer and all that goes with it overwhelms me. No, I cannot *handle cancer by myself.*

Another saying I have heard is, "If God brings you to it, He will bring you through it."

I've changed that to, "If God brings you to it, He can carry you through it."

No, I can't handle cancer by myself, but I don't have to.

Without a doubt, we knew that the Lord's love had carried us through the tough times and would continue to do so.

"DEHYDRATED" BUT IMPROVING

At Chris's three-week checkup on March 24, his blood tests showed he was dehydrated, although he was drinking 100 ounces of water a day to protect his kidney function. They wanted him to increase his water intake to 150 ounces per day. Other than sloshing to the bathroom frequently, he was already feeling better each day and could take deep breaths without coughing. He climbed stairs without getting terribly winded and had ridden his bike ten miles the previous Saturday.

We were ecstatic about his improved health from just a few months earlier.

A FATHER'S VOICE

We drove to Wichita Falls, Texas, on April 2 to surprise Shane at his collegiate bike race. That was the first race we had attended since Chris was diagnosed. When we arrived, he casually walked over to our son, who was bent over checking his tire pressure.

"Got enough air in there?" Chris asked.

At the sound of his father's voice, Shane jerked his head up. His eyes wide, his grin even wider, he threw himself at his dad, wrapping his arms around him. Surrounded by his teammates, we were all in tears. Shane's hero was back, enjoying life again.

As a bonus, Chris felt good enough to break out his camera and take photos of the races on Saturday and Sunday. He was a bit rusty but still got some good shots and had a blast doing something he loved. He was making another comeback.

Chris went for a bike ride on May 18 after he got home from work. After doing a couple of laps around our neighborhood, he realized he was breathing easier than on his previous rides. As he continued riding, he heard the same voice that had told him the previous year he was in for a long, hard battle.

But this time, the voice said, *The tumor is gone.*

ANOTHER GUINEA PIG

Chris had a brain MRI at MD Anderson. While sitting in the waiting room with another patient, they started talking about their cancer treatments. The other patient was getting an MRI as a follow-up after Gamma Knife.

"I had a two-millimeter brain tumor," the man said. "They told me the smallest tumor they had ever done before mine was three millimeters."

Chris smiled and raised his hand. "I'm the three millimeter."

Chris was so pleased. Because he took the chance to let them radiate his 3 mm tumor when the smallest they had done previously was 4 mm, they were willing to radiate an even smaller tumor to help this other patient.

NO EVIDENCE OF DISEASE

We were making trips to Houston every three weeks for checkups per the study protocol. Chris was seen by two research assistants, the physician's assistant (Cheryl), and the oncologist. Chris jokingly referred to them as his entourage.

At his twelve-week checkup for the clinical trial on May 26, 2011, there was no mention of the lung tumor in the radiologist's report. The scar tissue from the radiated brain tumor had completely resolved and was no longer visible. Chris asked if no mention of the lung tumor in the reports meant it was gone.

"You're considered to be in treatment with 'no evidence of disease' [NED]. In the world of advanced lung cancer treatment, that's as good as it gets," Cheryl said. "But NED doesn't necessarily mean the dead tumor is gone—it just means there's no evidence of active cancer."

You'd think we'd be jumping up and down with joy at this proclamation, but we weren't surprised. A voice had already leaked the news.

"Although you now have no evidence of disease, you will always be considered to have at least stable stage IV lung cancer and will need to be in active treatment for the rest of your life," she said. "Tiny diseased cells tend to hide. Advanced lung cancer almost always comes back."

I was unnerved to hear that he'd never be considered to be in remission, cured, or cancer-free. I suddenly realized this would be our new way of life.

"Will my lung reinflate?" Chris asked.

"It will probably never reinflate due to radiation fibrosis," Dr. Davis answered. "Performing radiation on any portion of the lung is essentially like removing that portion of the lung."

"We may have found the limits of medicine, but there's no limit to what God can do," Chris told me later.

His faith was stronger than mine. While I agreed that God *could* do such a miracle, deep down I had my doubts He *would*. I didn't tell Chris my doubts. I couldn't dash his hopes. Hope was the one thing that kept him going.

Going from death's door with stage IV lung cancer to NED, I realized God does His most magnificent work when the situation appears totally impossible from a human standpoint.

> *How can I repay the* Lord *for all His goodness to me?*
>
> —Psalm 116:12 NIV

Later that night, Chris wrote on CaringBridge:

> *The oncologist is very encouraged by the results. He said I can do whatever I feel like doing, and if it bothers me, don't do it again. I wish he had told me that a few weeks ago, because running the vacuum and doing the dishes has really been "wearing me down." At least that's my story, and I'm stickin' to it.*

BACK IN THE SADDLE

By June 16, Chris was finally back to his precancer weight, and his oxygen level was 99 percent. Riding his bike seemed to be helping. Tired of riding only ten miles at a time, he went for an endurance ride to see how far he could go. By the time he reached mile nine, he was out of energy. He briefly contemplated calling me to pick him up, but he felt if he gave up on himself, cancer would win one. He decided even if it took him all day, he'd finish the ride. He gritted his teeth and rode seventeen miles that day, big hills included. He proved to himself he may have cancer, but cancer didn't have him.

I was proud of Chris. He was fighting so hard to live.

LOSING FOCUS

Dr. Davis wasn't available at Chris's three-week checkup, so a different oncologist saw him.

"I don't know how long the crizotinib treatment will work," the doctor said, "but I guesstimate one to two years."

I knew she was telling us this based on the research studies, but I was fuming on the inside. *How dare she put a time limit on his treatment and dash his hope when he is doing so well on it!* I was sure Chris would be the exception.

He was already struggling with doubts that week because two friends weren't doing well with their lung cancer treatments and were experiencing complications. Another friend was losing his battle.

"You may get cancer out of your body, but you will never get it out of your mind." These were words spoken to us at our first Cancer Encouragement Group meeting. This is so true. Even though my husband was doing extremely well, he was still in a spiritual battle for his life. Doubts were beginning to creep in again, causing him to lose his focus on Jesus.

My focus, too, was blurred. I was wrapped in a mental fog. Life (and death) with cancer always played in my mind. It was like listening to four different songs at the same time on the radio. The softest was the one I wanted to hear, so I had to focus extra hard to hear it over the others. While doing bookkeeping at my client's office, I had to talk to myself silently to stay focused on the assignment. I was okay as long as I could hear my thought process for the data entry. But when other office conversations were louder than my thinking voice and mingled with the thoughts of cancer already plaguing my mind, it was a serious struggle to stay on task.

Many times when driving somewhere, I'd get to the stop sign at the end of our street and didn't know whether to turn left or right. I couldn't remember where I was going.

CRIZOTINIB RECEIVES FDA APPROVAL

Crizotinib was officially FDA approved on August 26, 2011, and was renamed Xalkori. Our medical team still referred to it as crizotinib, so we continued to call it that too. At the time, only two patients had a complete response to the drug (NED). Although we were never told, I assumed Chris was patient number two.

After the drug had received FDA approval, he continued in the study and received the drug for free. That was an answer to prayer. The price for a thirty-day supply was $9,600. Chris would be on this medication for the rest of his life—or as long as it was still effective.

We learned there was already a promising new drug called LDK378 in clinical trials to treat ALK mutations if the crizotinib quit working. We were thankful to know of a possible backup plan. God's timing is so good. In 2007, just three years before Chris was diagnosed, the ALK mutation hadn't been identified in lung cancer. Now they have successful treatments for it. What amazing progress in such a short time.

SPLASHING AND SLOSHING AROUND

September's extreme Texas heat prevented Chris from riding his bike, so we went to the neighborhood pool. Neither of us liked to swim, so it was purely for exercise. We swam across the short width of the pool, took a brief rest, and then swam back across, counting that as a lap. We did twenty-six laps before heading home. Occasionally, we had a contest like little children to see who could hold their breath the longest underwater. I usually won, but one night the guy with only one working lung tied with his wife, who had two good lungs. His good lung was getting stronger and was compensating for the bad one.

At Chris's last checkup, Cheryl had told him to increase his fluid intake by another 50–100 percent because his creatinine level still reflected that he was dehydrated.

"If your blood test shows 0.2 milligrams more elevation in the creatinine level, you could be kicked out of the clinical trial."

He kept records to prove he was following orders. He drank 136–178 ounces of water each day. Surprisingly, it only improved his creatinine level by 0.1 mg.

Concerned he could be dismissed from the clinical trial, I contacted Anne.

"He won't be kicked out," she assured me. "They won't dismiss him unless the medication no longer prevents the cancer from returning. If he acquires other medical issues, they will just try to help resolve them."

That was a huge relief.

CANCER DETECTION THROUGH BLOOD TESTS

Chris continued to be a guinea pig for cancer research, donating extra blood to help researchers find tumor markers for lung cancer. They were trying to detect the disease earlier through blood tests. Chris was determined that something good would come from his diagnosis, even if it only benefitted someone else.

> *"You intended to harm me, but God intended it for good to accomplish what is now being done, the saving of many lives."*
>
> —Genesis 50:20 NIV

Chapter 13

FRACTURED VERTEBRAE AND OSTEOPOROSIS

September 2011 was rough for Chris. He broke his little toe by stubbing it on a kitchen chair. Two weeks later, we went to Hawaii for a vacation, and he stubbed the same toe on a night stand in the dark. Things went downhill from there.

Before cancer, Chris didn't get easily stressed out, but after the diagnosis, he became quickly distressed over anything. His sense of direction, once good, now failed him on Oahu. He was so frustrated, he wanted to go back to the hotel and cancel our plans.

"I didn't come all the way to Hawaii just to spend our day in a hotel room," I said.

We managed to enjoy the beauty of the islands, but disaster struck at the airport on our way home. As Chris slung his camera backpack over his shoulder, he yelled in pain. I could tell he was in agony on the airplane, but he was stoic. By the time we got home, his back hurt whenever he would lie down, stand up, sit down, or just breathe. Then he came down with a cold. Each time he coughed or sneezed, he hurt even more. At one point, he sneezed hard, yelling in excruciating pain. It was difficult to watch him suffer.

"I want a 'do-over' for the month of September," he said. "Lord, what is the purpose of all this and for me having cancer?"

He didn't expect to get an answer. But six simple words flashed through his head.

So that God will be glorified.

He decided to pass on the do-over.

FRACTURED VERTEBRAE

In October, Chris had an MRI of his back. It revealed compression fractures at T5, T7, and T8. His spine was a ticking time bomb.

"This is something we would expect to find in someone much older with the beginning of osteoporosis," the doctor stated. "I haven't seen this before as a result of radiation, chemo, or the trial medicine." He was clueless as to why this happened.

Chris underwent a vertebroplasty procedure in November to repair his back. The doctor put small incisions on each side of the vertebra and then injected cement into the fractures to stabilize them. It was a day surgery and didn't even require stitches. Humpty Dumpty was put back together again. But the surgeon gave Chris bad news.

"You should never ride a bike again because it would be too hard on your back."

My husband was *not* happy. This news was almost as brutal as hearing, "You have lung cancer." At first, he felt he had beat the disease just to become a couch potato. But it provided the motivation he needed to complete physical therapy and develop the muscles around his spine so he could ride again.

SEVERE OSTEOPOROSIS, RECLAST, AND ONJ

We met with Dr. Camp,* an endocrinologist. She had no idea why Chris's vertebrae were fracturing and ordered tests to see why he had severe osteoporosis. None of the results provided a definitive answer, although a blood test showed that his testosterone was low.

"Over time, low testosterone can cause osteoporosis," she said.

We eventually found out why he developed the condition. In April 2012, a study discovered that crizotinib rapidly and significantly lowers testosterone in men, with 100 percent of the men in the study showing a rapid decrease in testosterone within days of starting the drug. Low testosterone reduces bone density, leading to osteoporosis.

Dr. Camp wanted to prescribe either a Reclast or Zometa infusion to help reverse his bone loss as quickly as possible so he wouldn't break a hip. "The most common side effects are flu-like symptoms," she said. She wanted him to have the infusion that day, but we stalled her until his next appointment.

I researched these two drugs after we got home to see if they would jeopardize Chris's health. I learned they are basically the same zoledronic acid drug given in different dosages. Reclast can cause anemia, and Chris was already anemic. It also can cause the femur—the strongest bone in the body—to break. But what I found next terrified me.

Reclast is a bisphosphonate drug known to cause osteonecrosis of the jawbone (ONJ)—death of the jawbone. Although rare, it had occurred in numerous patients, especially after invasive dental procedures. Chris and I cringed whenever we heard something was "rare" because he was always that rare patient. He had broken the crown on his tooth a couple of times, which caused me to worry. I saw photograph after photograph of people with ONJ, and it shook me to my core.

Zometa's website also stated that ONJ risk factors are higher in patients who are taking chemotherapy and corticosteroids. Chris was taking both.

My husband and I were amazingly compatible. I can't remember ever having a serious argument with him before in our first twenty-seven years of marriage. We were almost always on the same wavelength. Not this time. He felt he needed the Reclast infusion. My stomach was in knots at the thought of his getting it. I felt that if he consumed extra calcium and walked in the sunshine, it could build up his bones. We raised our voices in frustration over this to the point of tears, unable to come to an agreement on what to do. I sensed Satan was trying to tear us apart.

I wondered why the doctor didn't disclose this possible side effect so we could make an informed decision. *Does she expect Chris to die of lung cancer before he would have a chance to develop ONJ?* That thought upset me even more.

I went to work on Monday and confided to Lou Ann how terrified I was. She gave me words of wisdom I never forgot.

"There will probably come a day when Chris says he's had all the treatment he wants to endure. It's *his* body, and you will have to be prepared to respect his wishes. And because it is his body, you need to respect whatever decision he makes regarding his current treatment."

I went home that evening and prayed about what to do. It became clear to me. I sat with him on the living room couch. "Listen to me with an open mind regarding the information I found online," I said. "Then, if you still feel you should take the risk, I will respect your decision."

We prayed together about it afterward. He still felt he needed the treatment but would decide after talking with the doctor again.

"DeLayne the Researcher," as Chris called me, discovered that proton-pump inhibitor drugs such as Nexium and Protonix can cause osteoporosis in patients who are on the medication at high doses or for one year or longer. He had been on these drugs for years to treat acid reflux. In addition, I found the Symbicort corticosteroid inhaler prescribed for his lungs can lead to osteoporosis. I began to wonder if these drugs also contributed to his condition.

At our next appointment with Dr. Camp, I asked about Reclast's side effects. It's a patient's right to have full disclosure of risks before consenting to treatment. She merely repeated what she had told us before: "He might have flu-like symptoms for the first three days."

It wasn't until I specifically asked about ONJ that she admitted it was a possible side effect, but she downplayed the risk. The doctor said we always have to consider the risk versus the benefit of a treatment, and in his case, she felt the benefit strongly outweighed the risk.

Chris consented to the treatment. After he received the Reclast infusion, we were handed a printout of possible risks and side effects. Along with the warning for ONJ, it stated, "Men should not father a child while receiving this drug." It's a good thing we weren't planning to have any more children because no one advised us of this *before* the treatment.

I realized that even though we might have wonderful doctors, they were only human. Since they see so many patients, it must be challenging to remember what they have or haven't told someone.

Refusing to leave Chris's fate in the hands of the doctors, I learned as much about recommended treatments as possible so I could know what questions to ask at appointments. Knowledge was power and could have a profound effect on my husband's life.

A wise man is strong, and a man of knowledge increases power.

—Proverbs 24:5

Chapter 14

CAREGIVING

At a Cancer Encouragement Group meeting I attended without Chris, the survivors updated the group on their status. After I told how Chris was doing, the leader then asked, "How are you doing, DeLayne?" No one had ever asked me that. People would often ask Chris how he was doing with me standing right next to him, but it was as if I were invisible.

I was caught off guard by the question. I burst into tears, touched that someone cared about *me*. Someone understood I was suffering too. I later read an article regarding this phenomenon and became aware it would help me to discuss my feelings with other caregivers. I needed to talk with someone who understood what I was going through, but I didn't want to burden my husband. I couldn't let him know how worried I was or that his situation caused me stress.

Because of this, I helped start a group for caregivers at our church. Unfortunately, it had poor attendance. When caregivers need the group the most, it's difficult to leave the patient home alone. They put their own needs aside, sometimes to the detriment of their own well-being.

It reminds me of the emergency instructions given on an airplane. Passengers are to put their own oxygen masks on first before attempting to help someone else. It's not self-centered; it's the smart thing to do. If you were to pass out from lack of oxygen, you wouldn't be able to assist anyone. It's the same with being a caregiver. If you don't take care of your own needs—physical and emotional—you will be in no shape to successfully take care of anyone else.

I frequently played tug-of-war with my emotions. I tried to stay positive and be brave for Chris to give us both hope, but deep down I was a realist and knew I would need help sooner rather than later and possibly be facing widowhood. I was constantly thinking ahead. *What would I do if such and such happens? Who could I call to help me?*

While trying to control the negative thoughts constantly swirling in the back of my mind, I was also being stretched to my physical limits, taking on more of Chris's responsibilities at home. I took over the household chores we used to share plus the yard maintenance. That was in addition to working for clients, shopping, preparing meals, paying the bills, dealing with insurance paperwork, keeping track of which medical records I had requested and received, providing those records to his employer for intermittent disability requirements, attending all his appointments, and researching lung cancer treatments.

Sometimes it's as hard being the caregiver as being the patient. At least the patient is actively doing something to combat the disease. The one giving the care often feels helpless. That's why I became obsessed with research for clinical trials and tried to learn everything I could about the newest treatments for lung cancer. Keeping track of Chris's medical records and treatment history was another way I made myself feel useful. I obtained copies of every medical report and CDs of every scan. I took the most recent records with us to our local emergency room, since they didn't have online access to MD Anderson's system. This helped them quickly understand his condition and compare changes.

I read every word on the medical reports and looked up unfamiliar terminology. Knowing medical terms made understanding the doctors much easier and allowed me to ask appropriate questions. The doctors appreciated that I came prepared with questions.

I read about side effects of every medication Chris took and looked to see if he was prescribed drugs that shouldn't be taken together.

My husband's cancer consumed my time. But the love of my life was worth every second.

Be on your guard; stand firm in the faith; be men of courage; be strong. Do everything in love.

—1 CORINTHIANS 16:13–14 NIV

Chapter 15

PNEUMONIA, THORACENTESIS, AND A BROKEN VESSEL

On Thursday, December 29, 2011, Chris experienced an extreme case of chills with a bad headache, back pain, shoulder pain, fatigue, coughing, and vomiting. He ached all over. I had never seen him more miserable. He had difficulty standing because of the agonizing back pain. When his fever spiked to 102.3 degrees, I took him to the emergency room.

He received fluids and intravenous antibiotics, as well as morphine for his back. Within an hour, his pain level improved from an 8 to a 2. I was shocked at how easily he was able to pop out of the bed to go to the restroom an hour after taking the morphine. Tests showed he didn't have the flu, but it was possible he had a twenty-four-hour virus. It was difficult to tell from the x-rays whether or not he had pneumonia, so he was dismissed that evening with an oral antibiotic, just to be safe.

He hadn't had any appetite for three days and didn't want to drink much of anything. That wasn't good for someone who was supposed to drink 150 ounces of fluids a day. I finally started waking him up every thirty minutes on Friday to make him sip some water, Gatorade, or Sprite. Saturday afternoon I gave him a bath and washed his hair, since he hadn't had the energy to shower or bathe for three days. He apologized profusely that I had to do this for him.

PNEUMONIA

Chris spent New Year's Eve coughing so hard I was afraid he'd break another vertebra. He became breathless walking just fourteen steps from our bed to the bathroom. His lungs whistled when he breathed, and he had no energy. We didn't understand what was happening and were scared out of our wit.

I paged Dr. Davis, Chris's oncologist.

"Take him to the emergency room," he responded.

"Chris was in the ER two days ago," I explained, "and they sent him home on an antibiotic for possible pneumonia or a virus."

"You just need to give the antibiotic time to work or give the virus time to run its course," he said. So we stayed home.

Chris's temperature oscillated between normal and 102.6 degrees for the next three days. He refused to go back to the emergency room because he was finally able to keep some food and fluids down. Since his oncologist said we needed to give the antibiotic time to kick in, I didn't force Chris to go to the ER. I should have, but I was too medically naive and inexperienced to realize what was happening.

Nurse Anne called Monday morning, January 2, 2012. She heard we had paged Dr. Davis over the weekend and was following up. She suggested I take Chris to the ER or find a local oncologist to evaluate him that day. I spent several hours calling around to find a local doctor, with no luck. Either the offices were closed for the holiday, or they had no opening for a new patient that week. Since he was feeling a little better, we decided to wait until offices reopened.

Still unable to get an appointment the next day, I told Chris he needed to go to the emergency room. A short time later, I found him on his hands and knees, struggling to climb the stairs to his home office.

"What are you doing?" I asked.

"I've got work to do—I have to get these parts released today."

"We need to get ready to go to the ER!"

He stopped on the steps and buried his head in his arms in despair.

At that moment, Anne called to check on him. I told her how he was doing and that we hadn't been able to find a local oncologist.

"You need to get him to the ER," she said.

"He's refusing to go."

"Let me talk to him."

I handed the phone to Chris. He was curled up in a ball on the stairway, crying, as Anne talked to him. I don't know what she said, but she convinced him to go to the hospital. I give her credit for saving his life for the second time. The first time was getting him into the crizotinib study.

I had rarely seen my husband cry in our first twenty-seven years together. But that all changed with the cancer diagnosis. Facing a terminal diagnosis, not feeling good, being subjected to all sorts of torture time and time again, thinking of possibly leaving his loved ones behind, and being anxious about the pain he might have to endure wreaked havoc on his psyche.

We wanted to go where he would have the best care and the doctors would have his medical history, so we decided to drive the four and a half hours to Houston. I hurriedly packed for both of us while Chris took care of business from the kitchen table instead of upstairs.

The ER doctor wanted to prescribe Zofran for nausea. I consulted my trusty three-ring binder full of Chris's medical information, then said, "He's not allowed to have Zofran while taking crizotinib, as it can cause QTc prolongation." This is an abnormal heart rhythm that could suddenly stop his heart and be fatal. I handed the doctor a photocopy of a sheet Anne gave us listing medications he couldn't have with the clinical trial drug. He then prescribed a different drug that wasn't on the forbidden list.

Test results showed Chris had pneumonia and a lot of fluid around his lung. When the nurse came in to see him that evening, she asked an odd question.

"Did you have your right lung removed recently?"

"No."

Confused, she double-checked the patient's name on the computer and verified it was Chris's account. "It isn't visible on the x-ray."

He showed her his chest as proof he had no scars from lung surgery. She examined his back, too, as if she still didn't believe him. She pulled up the x-ray on the computer to show us, and sure enough, you couldn't see his right lung. The fluid was totally blocking the view.

THORACENTESIS

We finally moved to a private room on the heart/lung floor around 2:00 a.m. on January 4. The nurse checked on him every thirty minutes. We hoped to get a good nap later.

Anne called first thing in the morning. "Did you get him to the ER?"

"Yes, they admitted him to a room here last night."

"Here—as in MD Anderson?"

"Yes."

She was astonished that we drove all the way to Houston.

Chris gave me a big scare that morning. He coughed so hard, he ran out of air. He had a blank stare in his eyes as he gasped and fell backward onto his pillow, briefly passing out. For just a second, I thought his heart had stopped and he was dead. To my relief, he recovered quickly and opened his eyes.

The day soon became chaotic. Chris wasn't starving for attention. Everyone wanted to do something to him—often at the same time.

I was allowed to be with him as they performed a thoracentesis to drain the pleural effusion (fluid) from his lung. They offered to let me watch.

"No thanks. You'd have to pick me up off the floor."

I stayed in the procedure room but looked away as they inserted a needle into his lung through his back. I heard Chris groaning from the pain, and then they showed me the 1.75 liters of fluid from his lung. They couldn't get all the fluid since it was too painful for him to tolerate. I decided if he ever had to have that done again, I would *not* stay in the room.

He had a lot of pain that afternoon. After a dose of morphine, however, he felt much better.

"The staff is so good to me," Chris said. "I'm glad we drove to Houston after all."

Even with excellent care, I had to closely watch the medications prescribed. The doctors wanted to prescribe three different drugs that were on the forbidden list with his chemo pills. They said he really needed to take those medications, so he had to temporarily stop his chemo for seven to ten days to take the antibiotics.

Chris greatly improved after the thoracentesis. He received breathing treatments every six hours and did breathing exercises every hour. His sense of humor even came back.

I updated CaringBridge: "My man is a fighter and will win this battle too."

The hospital might as well have put a revolving door on Chris's room. We had so many doctors and nurses coming and going that it became laughable. We started guessing how long it would take for someone to walk in after he closed his eyes to take a nap. It was usually within zero to five minutes. Chris napped a total of fifteen minutes all day.

When I mentioned it to the nurse, she said, "You're here to get well, not to get rest."

I think that's their motto. I must admit though, he was getting wonderful care.

I was holding up better than I expected, but I had moments of sorrow. Besides seeing Chris suffering, I was sad because we were away from our boys again. Shane would be heading back to college before we returned home, and Chad wouldn't be at home much longer before traveling the globe with his cycling profession. We had lost precious time with them. I bawled when I realized we didn't get our traditional family photo in front of the Christmas tree. We weren't home on Christmas Day, and when we returned, Chris didn't feel well enough to want his photo taken. *What if that was his last Christmas?*

I remained emotionally strong the first two days. I was so physically and mentally exhausted by Thursday, though, I could barely pray. I tried to sleep in the fold-out bed next to my husband. Weeping silently, I couldn't form any cohesive thoughts other than, *Lord, please take away Chris's pain, help him breathe normally again, and restore his earthly body to his precancerous condition. You know my thoughts before they are formed, so You will just have to finish my prayer for me.*

> *In the same way the Spirit also helps our weakness; for we do not know how to pray as we should, but the Spirit Himself intercedes for us with groanings too deep for words; and He who searches the hearts knows what the mind of the Spirit is, because He intercedes for the saints according to the will of God.*
>
> —ROMANS 8:26

"A hospital is *not* a good place for sick people to be," Dr. Davis said the next morning. He dismissed Chris from the hospital on Friday, January 6, with instructions to return to the ER if he ran a fever of 100.5 degrees. We chose to stay in Houston over the weekend, since his health was still fragile and he had appointments scheduled for Monday at MD Anderson.

Chris ran a fever of 100.4 degrees at bedtime. We prayed it would improve overnight. I had napped only twenty minutes all week and was totally exhausted from lack of sleep. I failed to wake during the night to check on him.

A BROKEN VESSEL

I woke up eleven hours later and discovered Chris had a cold wash cloth on his neck, trying to bring his fever down.

"Did you take your temperature first?" I asked.

"No. Some things are better left unknown. I don't want to go back to the hospital." He was being stubborn again.

Later that morning, he wrote "A Broken Vessel."

> *Broken. That's what I am—broken. I can't remember at any point in my life being as broken as I am right now. I told one of the doctors that it's like all my dominoes were in a line, and someone walked up and pushed the first one. Now I'm powerless to stop them. Since mid-September, there's been one health issue after another. They have finally taken their toll.*
>
> *Physically, I'm exhausted. I'm not sure there's any part of my body that's working as it should. When it does work, it hurts. Just sitting up to eat or taking a short walk wears me out. Rolling over in bed takes tremendous effort. I try to not take many of the pain meds prescribed for me, but sometimes they're the only answer.*

Emotionally, I find myself becoming more disconnected each day. The doctor from Care Support told me it's okay to cry and would probably be good for me. I just thought, Dude, if I could, I would. *I feel like I have no control, and all the emotion has been sucked out of me.*

Mentally, I'm fatigued. I feel like I have pulled all-nighters for finals for the past week. Putting two thoughts together is becoming a real challenge. I do my best to just focus on each day and what it will take to get through it. With the string of bad days that I've had, it's hard to think of better days coming.

Spiritually, I've been drained. This is the area that most disturbs me. I try to read my Bible, but I just can't muster the desire. I try to pray, but all that will come out is, "God, please fix something!" Early one morning, I was lying in bed, pleading with God to show me some mercy. Suddenly, I realized the song "It is Well with My Soul" was playing in my head. I got mad and told God that under no circumstances was any of this well with my soul. Then I tried to recall some memory verses. The only verse that would come to mind was "MY GOD, MY GOD, WHY HAVE YOU FORSAKEN ME?" (Matthew 27:46). That pretty well summed up my feelings at that moment.

I still believe God is here, and He's working. I just wish I could feel Him more. I still believe something good will come from all of this. I just wish I could see it. I still believe that God is and will be glorified in all of this. I just wish He would get some glory somewhere else for a while.

Can God still use a broken vessel like me? I've read before that God saves His greatest work for His vessels after they've been broken and He's put them back together. I guess we'll see how He puts this one back together.

Be gracious to me, O Lord, for I am in distress; My eye is wasted away from grief, my soul and my body also. I am forgotten as a dead man, out of mind; I am like a broken vessel.

—Psalm 31:9, 12

Chapter 16

THE PATHWAY BACK

On Sunday, we decided some fresh air and sunshine might lift our spirits after walking through what felt like the valley of the shadow of death. We walked, hand in hand, three laps around the hotel parking lot. I also needed some perking up. I thought of the rays as the Son shining on my face, reminding me of the warmth of God's presence. His love beamed down on us, and I got recharged.

In Chris's post "The Pathway Back," he referred to what happened that day:

> *I was pretty well spent. I was uncertain as to how I would recover from all that had happened the previous week. I couldn't formulate a plan in my head and wasn't real impressed with where God's plan had me. It became evident that even though I wasn't particularly interested in spending time with God, He still wanted to spend time with me.*
>
> *The next morning, I turned on the TV and, out of habit, looked for Dr. Charles Stanley's show. I found him and was shocked to hear that day's message was about challenges to our faith. When he said all of us face failures in our faith sometimes, I about yelled, "Preach on, Brother!" He went on to make the point that God uses these tests as a means to*

increase and stretch our faith. I began to realize I was being stretched, and it wasn't very comfortable.

After Dr. Stanley finished, I flipped a few more channels and heard another familiar voice. I had stumbled onto Dr. David Jeremiah's broadcast. His message that day was on fighting discouragement. Really? *In the course of his message, he said all Christians will become discouraged. The only way to overcome deep discouragement is to read the Bible. Sometimes you'll be so discouraged that you'll have to force-feed yourself. He said you'll have to pray that God gives you verses of encouragement and that He sends you some encouragers.*

So on Sunday afternoon, I humbled myself and asked God to forgive me for my bad attitude. I asked for Him to give me some verses of encouragement and to send people to encourage me. When I opened my Bible, God provided verses that, once again, established that He was, is, and will forever be in control. He knows my situation better than I do. I simply have to trust His direction.

That evening, my sister called to encourage me and lift my spirits. Then I started receiving emails and comments on my blog. People were thanking me for being honest about my battle, and they told me they'd be praying for me. Two days later, a woman I've never met left a comment for me about how my latest blog entry had helped her and her mother understand what another family member was going through. Even in my brokenness, God was still building.

These last two weeks, I've still had to force-feed myself some days. But at least I'm now on the pathway back.

Our troubles were teaching us to lean heavily on God's grace. Our hope wasn't only for our immediate future but also for our eternal future. No matter what suffering we faced in this life, because we accepted the Lord as our personal Savior, we had the assurance of spending eternity with Him.

Chris and I said so many times, "I don't know how people who don't know the Lord can deal with something like cancer."

PARTNERING WITH THE NURSE

On January 9, we saw the oncologist per the clinical trial protocol. We also spent a lot of time with Anne.

"Listen to your body and get to the emergency room if you need to. If you're oxygen deprived and your brain doesn't comprehend the seriousness of your condition, listen to your wife," she jokingly scolded Chris. Then she turned to me. "If you feel Mr. Haga needs to go to the emergency room and he refuses to go, call 911, and they'll send someone to assess him. If they deem he needs to go to the ER, they'll take him."

It had never occurred to me to call 911. How could I have missed something so simple?

Chris stopped taking crizotinib temporarily while on antibiotics for the pneumonia because the combination of the drugs could stop his heart. Anne didn't know how many doses of crizotinib he could miss and still stay in the study. I silently panicked at the news. That was his lifeline.

Anne had become more than just a nurse. She partnered with us to help him in any way possible. I privately sent her emails about what Chris was or wasn't doing that he shouldn't or should be doing. I told her when he was depressed. She convinced him to talk with a professional about his situational depression. During our appointments, she would ask Chris how he was doing. Then she would look to see if my facial expression agreed with his answer or reflected he wasn't being honest. Anne then got him to confess the truth. She treated my input as valuable.

Before we left, we discussed Chris's NED status.

"You're a rare case," she told him. "God apparently had a hand in your healing." She then warned Chris it may take weeks or months to recuperate fully from this episode.

He took that as a challenge. That day, we walked from one end of MD Anderson to the other. Although he was extremely fatigued and walked slowly, he refused to use a wheelchair.

WRESTLING WITH SATAN

Chris finally felt up to going to church with me on January 22, but as he was getting ready, I noticed he had to rest frequently. He described what happened in "Wrestling with Satan."

> *During the previous two weeks, I started to spiritually find my way back and physically improve. I was tired of walking around the block and started walking the mile around the neighborhood. My breathing exercises showed real improvement.*
>
> *I hadn't been able to attend church for several weeks. After this last stint in the hospital, I've been afraid of being in large groups of people, especially during the peak flu season. However, I knew I needed to be back in the body for worship.*
>
> *After I got up Sunday morning and had breakfast, I did my first round of breathing exercises and saw the best early-morning results yet. I thought that was a good sign to start getting ready for church. However, after taking my shower, I noticed I was extremely short of breath. I also noticed my back was beginning to hurt worse. I started to doubt I'd be able to get out of the house. Sitting on the bed trying to catch my breath, I asked why, all of a sudden, this was such a battle.*
>
> *That's when I heard my little voice say,* Satan doesn't want you in church. *Moving a little slower but with more determination, I continued to get ready for church. I could tell the wrestling match wasn't going to end.*

After parking at church, we had a couple of hundred yards to walk to the entrance. The closer we got, the harder each step became. This was a much shorter walk than I've been doing, but, with each of the final few steps, I was saying, "Help me, Jesus." Once I was in the church, I noticed that I was breathing hard, but my feet and legs felt lighter. I was able to make my way into the sanctuary, sit down, and begin catching my breath. I had made it to church.

After the service, I knew why Satan wrestled with me every step to church. Once again, the service was filled with hymns that contained words I needed to hear. The sermon was from Psalm 139 about how God had put me together. He knew the plans He had for me and that only He knew the number of my days. Satan didn't want me to be encouraged. He doesn't want me back in the game.

But, thanks to Jesus, Satan has lost another match.

You might be wondering, *If God already determined the number of our days before we were even born, then why bother with treatments?*

It's our responsibility to do what we can to increase the quality of our life until our time is up. Doctors and medicine are gifts from God that He provides to extend lives to the day He has chosen. We chose to seek the best medical care while praying for His will.

Chris continued to improve and playfully *chased* me up two flights of stairs at the hotel a week later. Although life for him would never be normal again, he was feeling more like his old self.

My times are in Your hand; deliver me from the hand of my enemies and from those who persecute me.

—Psalm 31:15

Chapter 17

A NEW LEASE ON LIFE

Our hopes for improvement were dashed again as the roller coaster continued. A CT scan showed Chris fractured his T9 vertebra, probably from coughing hard. The L2 also had a defect that could cause it to fracture. He had another vertebroplasty on March 9 to repair his spine.

"Don't do anything that strains or jerks your back, or you'll need surgery again. If you ride a bike, be very careful that you don't fall, or you could fracture your back," the surgeon told him.

We were flabbergasted the doctor even mentioned Chris might ride his bike again. He realized Chris needed something to look forward to doing when he got better.

We saw the surgeon six weeks later for a follow-up. He was astonished Chris was no longer taking morphine for pain and that he had only used half a dose of the 15 mg prescribed. The doctor was pleased with Chris's progress.

"You can start riding your bike again if you will be extremely careful," he said.

My husband's eyes lit up. He had just received a new lease on life.

By June 19, his breathing exercises had greatly improved, reaching 3,750 on an incentive spirometer, a plastic device that measures lung capacity when taking a deep breath. It also exercises and strengthens the lungs. We were told that an average healthy person can reach 2,000.

Chris rode his bike a total of forty miles that week. He was making great strides.

RISK OF QTC PROLONGATION

Dr. Heymach filled in for Dr. Davis at the next checkup. We thanked him for suggesting Chris be tested for the ALK mutation, and I gave him credit for saving my husband's life. The doctor saw that not only was Chris alive, he had most of his quality of life back.

Chris's local urologist wanted to prescribe a medication to prevent kidney stones, but it could cause QTc prolongation. I asked Dr. Heymach what the risk of sudden death was if Chris took that medication while on crizotinib.

"It's not worth the risk," the doctor replied.

I mentally noted how quickly he answered the question as to the severity of the risk.

PIPELINE

In June, we found out Chris was the last patient still in the study for crizotinib at MD Anderson. All the others had dropped out due to progression of disease. We also learned other ALK inhibitor medicines were already in the pipeline. That meant if crizotinib became ineffective for him, there were other potential treatments available.

Let my soul live that it may praise You.

—Psalm 119:175

Chapter 18

GOD CLOSES AND OPENS TWO DOORS

Chris was so unhappy with his job he wanted to take early retirement and enjoy the rest of his life as long as possible.

As much as I knew he wanted to leave, we needed his health insurance. It would be hard for him to find another job because of his age. It would be even harder battling stage IV lung cancer. There could be a waiting period before new insurance would cover a preexisting condition. Because Chris was doing so well, he might possibly live for a long time. If he left his job and lost his income, medical insurance premiums could be very expensive. Medical bills could ruin us financially.

It would be challenging for me to find a full-time job because I needed to take off work to go with Chris to appointments and take care of him when he was hospitalized. I just couldn't give him the okay to retire early.

As he left for work on August 8, Chris leaned against the door to the garage, crying, totally despondent. I felt so bad for him, and my heart was breaking. If I had suggested he quit his job, he would have jumped at the opportunity. But he trudged to work every day to provide for his family. That's sacrificial love.

DOOR NUMBER ONE

Just a week later, Chris learned his department no longer existed. He would have thirty days to find another job within the company or be laid off. God was taking the matter into His own hands.

"If this happened two years ago, I would have been upset," Chris said. "Although I'm not happy about it, when I think about all God has done and provided the past two years, I believe He can handle this situation as well."

I looked at it as an opportunity to figure out if God wanted Chris to continue working or retire. If he was unable to find another job, then maybe God was saying it was time to take early retirement. If God provided another job, Chris was supposed to continue working.

In my mind, if he got another job, that meant he would be healthy enough to work for a long time. I was praying for a job for him for more than one reason.

He had three interviews with the Quality Assurance department. Just a week before the deadline for being laid off, he was offered a job with the Medical Device group, which sells chips that go in the PET scans, CT scans, MRIs, and ultrasounds. God works in mysterious ways. Chris suddenly had a vested interest to make sure that Texas Instruments made quality products.

TWO LIVING MIRACLES AT LUNCH

In mid-September, Chris pulled 4,000 on the incentive spirometer. That's as high as the scale reads. He also swam twenty laps at our neighborhood pool with more ease than I did. I was amazed at his continued improvement.

By December 6, he weighed 15 pounds more than his normal weight. Anne had told him previously, "The more weight you can keep on, the better. It means you're healthy."

He took her word for it and added a little extra for insurance.

After his appointment, we ate lunch with our friends Brett and Heather Crombie in the MD Anderson cafeteria. A mutual friend back home had asked us to mentor them, and we created our own little support group when we were in Houston. Brett, also diagnosed with lung cancer, was doing great after a scary Thanksgiving week in which he had emergency brain surgery. The cancer had metastasized to the lining of his brain, and the doctors told his family he might not make it. Yet two living miracles were sitting across the table from each other, chatting away.

PICKING UP BREAD CRUMBS

On December 21, 2012, Dr. Green* examined Chris at MD Anderson for the trial protocol since Dr. Davis wasn't available. The oncologist said a suspicious spot in Chris's lung had grown from 1.6 cm to 2 cm. They scheduled a PET scan at his next checkup in January to better understand what was going on. If the spot was cancer, Chris would have to stop taking the inhibitor drug he had been on for the past twenty-two months because it was no longer effective. He wasn't showing any signs of the spot being malignant, other than losing 5 pounds in less than a month, and he was trying to be upbeat about the situation. But I quietly panicked whenever he started losing weight.

Chris was mentally preparing himself for what the PET scan might reveal as he wrote "Picking Up Bread Crumbs."

> *From the beginning, we were informed there was no assurance of how long the medicine would work. I've done my best to push those thoughts out of my mind. Beating lung cancer once is hard enough. Beating it twice would be more difficult. When you're fighting cancer, you focus on the present and not what you may have to face tomorrow. However, now I have to begin thinking about what may lie ahead. Is there yet another bend in the road in this quest to beat the disease?*

In seeking to look ahead, I find myself spending more time in the past. I keep replaying these last two and a half years. They've been nothing short of an incredible miracle. I've taken the medicine for twice as long as the average patient in any of the trials. I've accomplished things that have the doctors shaking their heads and making statements like, "You're not typical."

As good as that may be, I still feel like I've missed something. I feel like maybe the disciples did in John 6. Jesus performed an incredible miracle by feeding over five thousand people with five loaves of bread and two small fish. Once everyone was fed and satisfied, Jesus told the disciples to go pick up the leftovers. He told them to let nothing go to waste. I don't think He was only talking about the food. I think Jesus wanted them to see with how much abundance He had met their needs.

As I've been reflecting on these past two and a half years and picking up the bread crumbs, there's one thing I'm seeing consistently: Jesus has been far ahead of us the whole time. He's known from the beginning what was to come and laid the stones for us to walk on. He knows what the results of the PET scan will be and is already preparing the path we will take.

PLANNING AHEAD

Back at MD Anderson, the PET scan showed activity in the previously radiated area. On Thursday, January 10, 2013, Chris had a needle biopsy to determine if it was cancer.

God was the pilot in charge of this trip, but I wasn't willing to be just a passenger. I intended to be a co-pilot. But I had a lot of learning to do to earn those wings, so I got busy. This team approach was crucial for Chris as I resolved to continue helping him fight for his life.

While sitting at his bedside in the recovery room after the biopsy, I researched clinical trials on my laptop. My head spun from the myriad of options. Feeling overwhelmed with lack of direction and so many statistics to comprehend on the success rate of each drug, I prayed for God to lead me to the right trial and to close the door to ones that wouldn't be the best choice.

The previous year, Chris found a local oncologist in Dallas for emergencies. Dr. David Gerber at UT Southwestern had many patients on crizotinib, so we knew we were in good hands. At an appointment in August 2012, I had asked Dr. Gerber what drugs were available for the ALK mutation if crizotinib quits working.

"LDK378 and an HSP90 drug are available, but they're so new, it's unknown how long they'll work." At the time, the nearest trial for LDK378 was in Denver.

In my research on January 10, 2013, I read that LDK378 trials were showing an 80 percent positive response rate, so it was our preferred choice. Unfortunately, I couldn't find any of those trials open in the United States. All their phase I trials were closed, and phase II hadn't opened.

Fayetteville, Arkansas—a five-hour drive—was the closest place with the HSP90 drug, which showed a 60 percent positive response rate.

Chris and I had decided we didn't want to go up north where the winter weather was unpredictable. Flying anywhere wasn't a feasible option either. We couldn't depend on airlines to be on schedule, and being in an airplane while dealing with lung cancer and side effects of treatment wouldn't be a pleasant experience for anyone on board. Health concerns were also an issue with many people carrying germs in a compact space. Traveling would require extra time away from work, and it would be expensive to fly every few weeks. Plus we'd have no support system so far from home. We agreed to seek treatment in Arkansas unless Dr. Davis gave us a better option closer to home.

After chest x-rays confirmed Chris's lung hadn't collapsed from the biopsy and he didn't have pneumonia, he was dismissed from recovery. Thirty minutes later, we met with Dr. Davis, and I asked my preplanned questions.

"Which new clinical trial drugs are most promising for ALK?"

The doctor shrugged. "I don't know. We don't have anything else here yet for ALK."

"Which new drugs are coming to MD Anderson?" I asked.

"I don't know."

I was checking off my questions faster than expected. "Is it better to go with the standard chemo Alimta or wait for a clinical trial?"

"I'd recommend you find a clinical trial at either Massachusetts General in Boston or at UCLA in California."

"You're not much help," I said, half joking. I was disappointed he didn't take a stronger role in guiding us to the next treatment. *What if I hadn't already done research and found the trial in Fayetteville?*

Chris spoke up. "We've decided on the HSP90 trial in Arkansas."

"Okay. I'll make the call to get things rolling," Dr. Davis said as he walked out the door. We all presumed the biopsy would show the cancer had returned.

We discovered the doctors at major cancer centers don't solely treat patients. Most are also teaching, researching, and helping develop more effective treatments. The world of medicine is constantly and rapidly changing. There are countless kinds of a disease. With treatments frequently improving, even the most brilliant doctors can't keep current on every new finding. They tend to specialize in specific areas, such as within subtypes and mutations of lung cancer. Even if they could know everything about all treatments offered, the information would quickly be outdated. That's why I found it important to be actively involved with searching for the most current and effective treatments available.

PNEUMONIA AND THORACENTESIS

Things can change quickly when lung cancer is involved. Four hours after x-rays showed Chris didn't have pneumonia, he developed a 102.3-degree fever. I took him to the emergency room, where he was admitted to the hospital—with pneumonia. I found out later from medical records his score for mortality risk was level four due to his condition. There are only five levels.

Friday afternoon, doctors attempted a thoracentesis to drain the pleural effusion from around his lung. The procedure was halted when Chris's blood pressure dropped to 77/55. An ultrasound showed that although there was a large amount of fluid, it was loculated, which meant it was contained in numerous smaller sacs. If they were to insert the tap, the only fluid drained would be from the sac they tapped.

"There's nothing we can do to drain the fluid," the doctor said.

Chris asked friends and family to pray for divine intervention for the fluid to reduce.

CONTRAINDICATION

The nurse came in at noon on Saturday to dispense two antibiotics prescribed by Dr. Green, the oncologist assigned to the hospital shift that weekend. I'd never heard of Avelox before, so I questioned the nurse.

"Could it cause QTc prolongation? Chris can't have antibiotics that can cause that condition while he's taking crizotinib because they could stop his heart."

He had taken his chemo medication three hours earlier and needed it twice daily.

Chris was exasperated with me. "Don't worry—if Dr. Green prescribed it, it must be okay to take. He knows I'm on crizotinib."

"Please wait until we get clarification that it's safe to take," I pleaded.

Despite my objection, Chris swallowed the antibiotics.

I immediately did a Google search for Avelox. My first search showed it caused QTc prolongation, and then I also found it on the drug information sheet the nurse had handed me. Totally freaking out, I called the nurse back in. Crying and shaking, I told her what I had discovered. "Please contact the pharmacy and ask about the safety of taking these two drugs together."

The pharmacist discovered I was right, and the doctor switched the prescription to a safe antibiotic. They performed an EKG and made sure Chris's heart was okay.

The doctor may not have known about the contraindication since crizotinib was an investigational drug.

The next day, we asked Dr. Green's opinion on the next best viable cancer treatment for Chris, since he was knowledgeable of the studies for ALK at MD Anderson.

"I'd recommend targeted therapy such as X-396, if it's available, or immunotherapy. The clinical trials won't be available here for at least a couple more months, though. You could also try other clinical trials or standard chemo."

"What are the side effects of HSP90?" I asked, since that's what we were planning.

"Don't worry about side effects in the grand scheme of things. It's more important to get rid of the cancer even if the treatment causes adverse side effects."

"Since the pleural effusion can't be drained, are there other options?" I asked.

"No."

"Will it go away on its own?"

"No. If we were to try to drain each tiny pocket of fluid, it would make it worse. Many times, the pockets will divide into smaller pockets when poked."

That was discouraging news since Chris was having more trouble breathing.

He was dismissed from the hospital. Although he was feeling better physically, we were both mentally whooped. We spent the night at a nearby hotel, as Chris was nervous about going home for fear he would start running a fever again and end up in the emergency room. Despite the recent frustrations, MD Anderson was our security blanket.

DOOR NUMBER TWO

We headed home from Houston on Monday and stopped to grab a hamburger for lunch. Chris's phone rang as I pulled into the parking lot. It was the research assistant from Highlands Oncology Group in Fayetteville, Arkansas.

"I'm calling to introduce myself and confirm we're working on getting you into the clinical trial here in case the biopsy shows the cancer has returned," Amanda Sisemore said.

"Is this for the HSP90 trial?" Chris asked, holding the phone out so I could hear the conversation.

"No. That trial just closed. This is for the LDK378 phase II trial that just opened."

A wave of relief came over us, and we felt the warmth of tears. This was the answer to our prayers. It was possible Chris could win the battle with that drug as ammunition.

Looking back, we eventually realized the delay in his original diagnosis in 2010 allowed God's perfect timing for future treatment as soon as it became available. He closed the door to one trial and opened the door to the next chemo that was best for Chris. God was still navigating our course.

When would we learn to trust His timetable?

"Ask and it will be given to you; seek and you will find; knock and the door will be opened to you. For everyone who asks receives; he who seeks finds; and to him who knocks, the door will be opened."

—Matthew 7:7–8 NIV

Chapter 19

SECOND CLINICAL TRIAL

We received the pathology results on January 15. As suspected, it was positive for recurrent cancer. Admittedly, we were a bit down, but God had already reassured us He had things under control.

Two days later, we met with Dr. Gerber at UT Southwestern and discussed LDK378. He said they hoped to get the trial open there in the next three weeks, but it could take longer. We didn't feel we could wait and wanted to begin treatment as soon as possible, even if it meant driving to Arkansas.

We were ecstatic to be getting in a phase II trial. Here's why:

Phase I participants start at a very low dose of the experimental drug. As more participants join, it's increased for each new group until the most effective dose is found or a toxic level is reached. A patient may get a dose that is too low to work or so strong it's toxic to the body.

Phase II gives the drug at the best dose determined during phase I, and it's used to determine how effective the drug is.

Phase III frequently randomly selects who gets the trial drug and who gets a placebo or standard treatment for comparison.

We arrived at Highlands Oncology Clinic in Arkansas on January 22. The clinicians were on Chris "like a duck on a June bug." As soon as he sat down, they called him to the exam room.

Amanda went over the clinical trial consent form with us. "Novartis [the drug manufacturer] has been calling me all morning to see if you have consented to the trial yet. You will be the first person in the United States and the third person in the world to enter this phase II trial."

This was an exciting time in the advancement of lung cancer treatment, and Chris would help pave the way for future patients to get an extended lease on life.

Sometimes a visit to the doctor's office felt like landing in a foreign land. We were scared, alone, and surrounded by a language we didn't understand. But the people we encountered through each portion of our trip enriched us through the relationships we formed.

As I sat in the waiting room while he got more scans, Amanda saw me and sat down to chat.

"We were so grateful the day you called and said the HSP90 trial had been closed but the LDK378 trial had just been opened," I said. "We felt God wanted Chris in this trial and had made it possible." We both teared up, our hearts filled with gratitude, and she gave me a warm hug. I knew Chris and I would be at home there.

Next, we met with the oncologist, Dr. Eric Schaefer. We were immediately impressed with him. He read through Chris's records before meeting with us, and he accurately repeated the health history, types of treatments, and dates of treatments from the last two years—by memory. He was up on the ALK mutation and drugs used to treat it. He even gave us his personal cell phone number. The doctor appreciated my list of questions and was surprised when I had answers to his questions from documentation at my fingertips.

Dr. Schaefer was optimistic. "Based on the way you responded to crizotinib," he told Chris, "I think you'll respond just as well to this new treatment."

Chris had to be off the old medication for seven to ten days before starting the new drug. They refer to that as a "washout period." It's to ensure results are from the new drug and not the former treatment.

By the time we left Fayetteville, it was evident this was where God wanted us. Amanda said only 137 participants would be asked to be in the study from around the world. What are the odds that less than an hour before meeting with the oncologist in Houston, I would find the only place in the United States that had opened phase II recruiting for the LDK378 clinical trial we needed in a tiny, unknown clinic? It was more than coincidence that the trial opened just as Chris's medicine stopped working. The puzzle pieces fell into place in God's impeccable timing.

Three days later, Amanda called me at home and said, "Before Chris can enter the clinical trial, Novartis needs documentation from a biopsy proving he has the ALK gene. Can you have the hospital send the pathology report to me as soon as possible?"

"I can do better than that. I have a copy of the pathology report right here in my files. I'll fax it to you in a few minutes."

Cutting out the middleman prevented a possible delay in treatment.

Back at the Arkansas clinic five days later, we felt an air of excitement. Amanda handed Chris his first dose of LDK378. On January 30, 2013, he officially became the first person in the United States to start the phase II clinical trial.

"I've just been praising the Lord all morning for this," Amanda said.

"So have we!" we chimed in unison.

Be still, and know that I am God.

—Psalm 46:10 NIV

Chapter 20

FROM RAGING FEVER TO HEALTH

Dr. Gerber was keeping tabs on Chris in Dallas and referred him to a pulmonologist to address the lung fluid buildup. The specialist discussed various invasive and unappealing procedures that could be done. Chris elected to do nothing, as he didn't have peace about any of the options. He prayed the Great Physician would perform a miracle and make the loculated pleural effusion simply disappear.

Dr. Gerber reexamined Chris on February 7 to check on a blood clot in his leg. His temperature spiked to 102.3 degrees twenty minutes after arriving. After blood cultures and chest x-rays didn't find a cause, he went home with an antibiotic. An hour later, his temperature soared to 103.6.

I called UT Southwestern, and the triage nurse told me to take him to the emergency room.

"Chris doesn't want to go," I said.

"He could have a raging infection called sepsis," said the nurse. "We are the boss of him in this instance."

Hearing the urgency in her voice, I determined Chris was going, even if I had to drag him. But tests at the hospital couldn't find anything wrong, so they gave him intravenous fluids and sent him home.

SHOWING IMPROVEMENT

During the first two weeks on the trial drug, Chris lost 7 pounds due to the cancer, nausea, and intestinal cramping the drug caused. He gained back almost 5 pounds by his first monthly follow-up visit in Arkansas. As Chris's health overall was improving, Dr. Schaefer wanted to hold off on treating the pleural effusion.

"I want to see if the medication will help it resolve," he said.

During March, Chris felt well enough to make repairs on our shed, play catch with Shane like old times, take a walk, and fix sprinkler heads in the yard. He even raked our entire large yard of thatch—not an easy task for a *healthy* person. It improved his spirits to feel helpful around the house and do normal activities again.

He was able to pull 3,750 on the incentive spirometer—improved from 3,000 a month earlier. His breathing sounded peaceful when he slept. I stayed awake just to listen to him breathe. It was comforting and reassuring to hear him breathing deeply and in rhythm with my own.

After eight weeks in the clinical trial, CT scans showed the cancer was shrinking and the pleural effusion was improving. But we already knew that based on how Chris was feeling.

A month later, he swam twenty laps at the hotel pool, walked more than a mile at Lake Fayetteville, and walked uphill at Devil's Park. He was well on his way to being healthy again.

> *"For I know the plans I have for you," declares the* Lord, *"plans to prosper you and not to harm you, plans to give you hope and a future."*
>
> —Jeremiah 29:11 NIV

DREAMS INTERSECT

Injuries prevented our son Chad from racing at the end of the previous season, leaving him discouraged and frustrated while recuperating.

Chris said battling cancer was hard, but watching his son struggle was even harder. He wondered if he had offered Chad good advice to pursue his dream of becoming a pro cyclist.

In the meantime, Chris was still pursuing his own dream to be cancer-free. His routine exam for the trial went well on Tuesday, but we hung around Fayetteville for five more days.

When God opened the door to the study in Arkansas, we couldn't figure out why, of all the clinics in the United States that were trying to open the trial, this little clinic was first.

When Chad found out his team, Optum, would be in the Joe Martin Stage Race in Fayetteville the week of Chris's exam, we extended our stay. This was the first time we would see our son race as a professional.

Chad won the race—his first National Racing Calendar win.

Here's an excerpt from Chris's blog post "When Dreams Intersect."

> *After seeing Chad cross the finish line, I let out a big yell, saw his team director, and gave him a hug. I then started toward the team van where I knew Chad would be. Chad caught up to me about halfway there. He gave me a big hug and said, "That was for you. I love you and am so glad you're here to see it."*
>
> *Then I knew that there, in downtown Fayetteville, God had allowed our dreams to intersect. Chad is a pro cyclist and, if even for just that moment, I was healed of cancer.*

> *At Gibeon the LORD appeared to Solomon during the night in a dream, and God said, "Ask for whatever you want me to give you."*
>
> —1 KINGS 3:5 NIV

NO EVIDENCE OF DISEASE AGAIN

Chris ran a fever about every four to six weeks, so Dr. Schaefer prescribed an antibiotic to keep on hand to avoid another trip to the ER. It did the trick.

At his sixteen-week checkup, scans showed two tumors were gone, and one was barely visible. The fluid on his right lung was also reducing. Thanks to a divine intervention, no treatment to drain the fluid would be necessary.

Chris and I had adapted to our new routine of monthly trips to Arkansas and had started taking his disease status for granted. But on June 23, we received a stark reminder of the enemy we were up against when our friend Brett lost his battle age at thirty-seven. That drove Chris to fight the disease for the two of them. He continued to ride his bike and improve.

He again ran a high fever after a brain MRI and CT scan of his chest, abdomen, and pelvis. The fever disappeared the next morning.

On July 16, 2013, Dr. Schaefer declared Chris to have no evidence of disease. This was the second time in three years God had given us that miracle. Although we suspected that's what the scans would reflect, we were grateful for the official confirmation.

Only 50 percent of lung cancer patients survive longer than one year after diagnosis. Had we asked the doctors three years earlier what the chances were that Chris would live to see Shane graduate, the odds wouldn't have been good. But those are the statistics of man—not the plans of God. By God's grace, Chris was beating the odds.

Shane graduated from Texas A&M University in August, and Chris was able to see our younger son walk across the stage to get his diploma.

For Your righteousness, O God, reaches to the heavens,
You who have done great things; O God, who is like You?

You who have shown me many troubles and distresses will revive me again, and will bring me up again from the depths of the earth. May You increase my greatness and turn to comfort me.

—Psalm 71:19–21

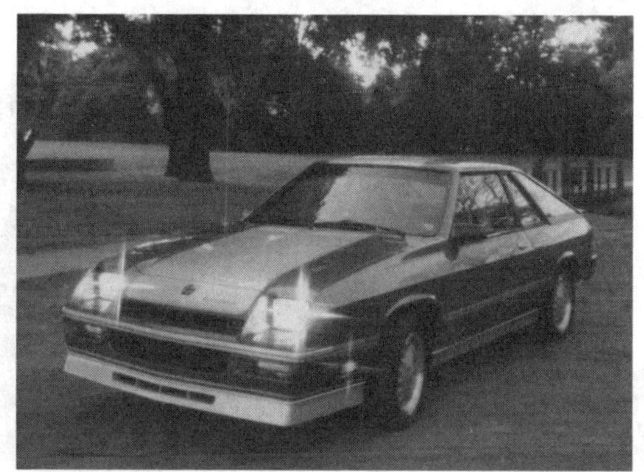

The car that brought us together, July 1983

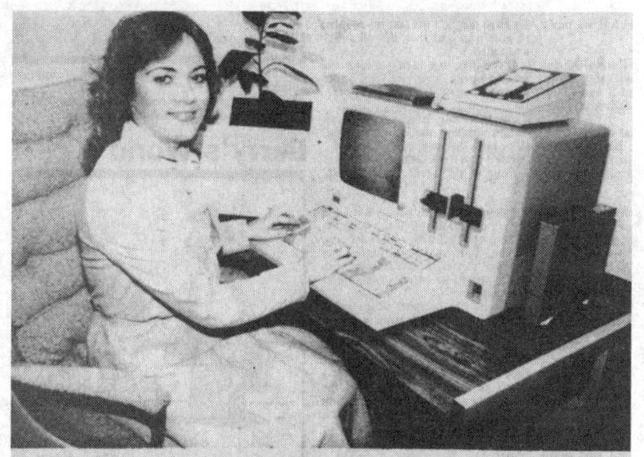

The newspaper ad involved in the joke, fall 1983

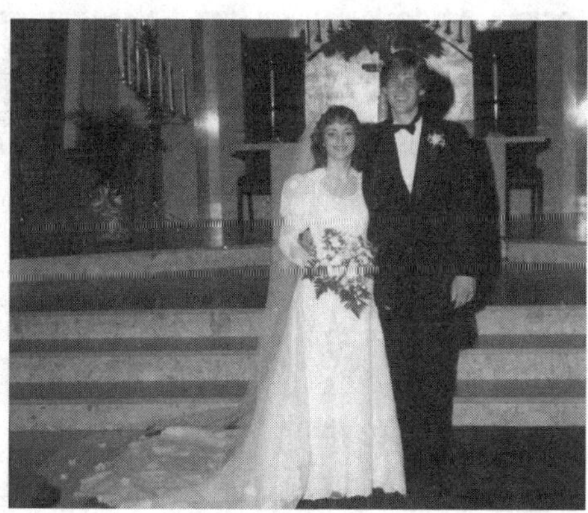

July 7, 1984

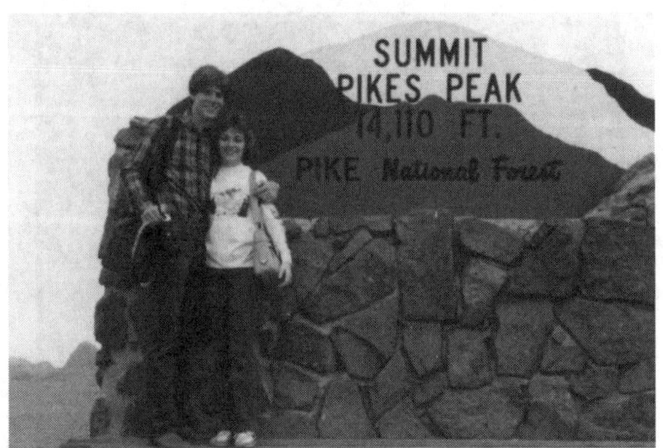

Honeymoon in Colorado Springs, July 1984

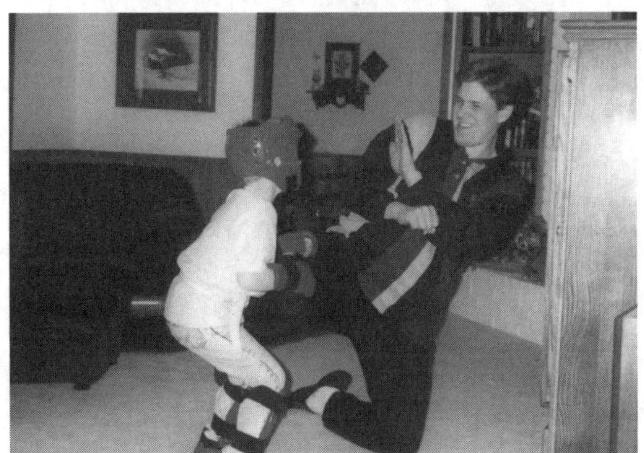
Sparring with Chad, 1995

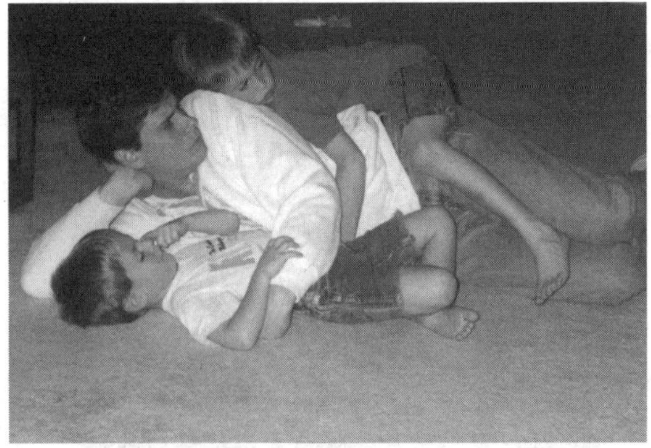
Snuggle time watching TV, 1995

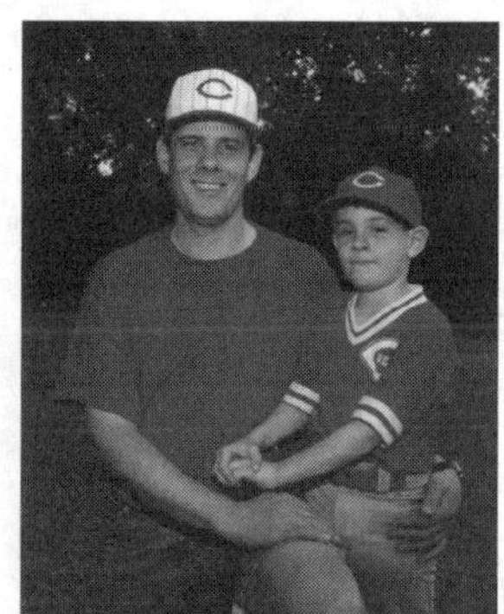

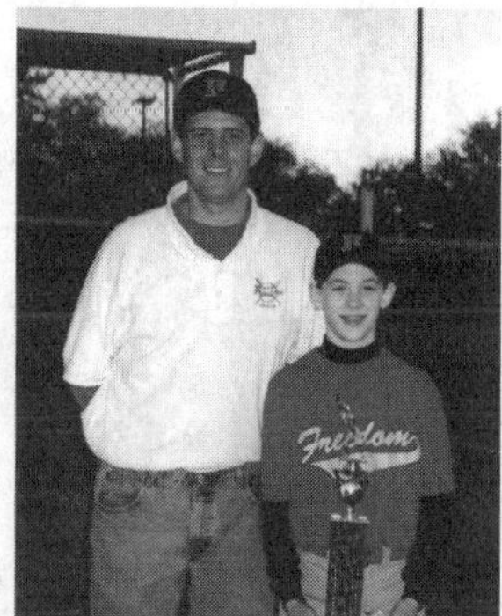

(Left) Coach Dad and Shane, 1998
(Right) Coach Dad and Chad, 2000

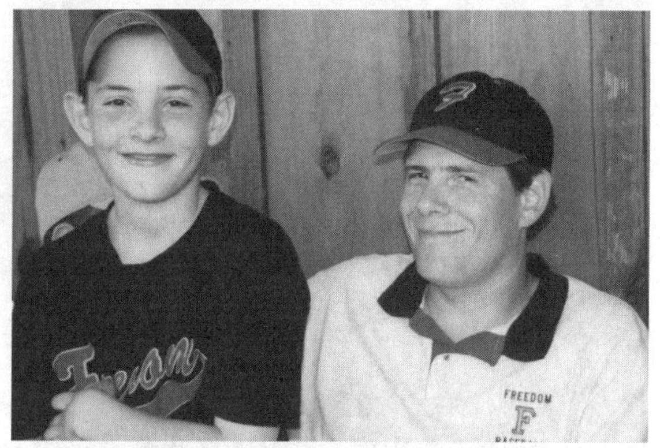

Shane and Coach Dad, 2002

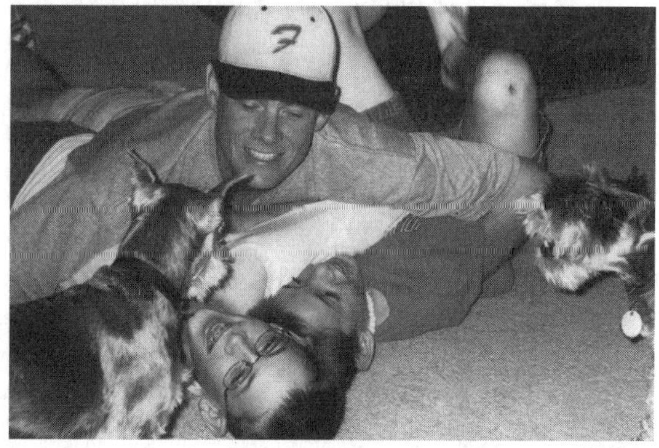

Typical wrestling/tickling match
(dogs are cheerleading), 2002

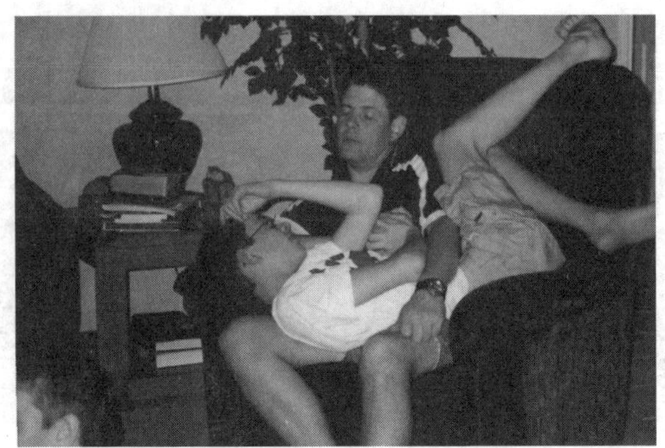

Father/son chat with Chad, 2003

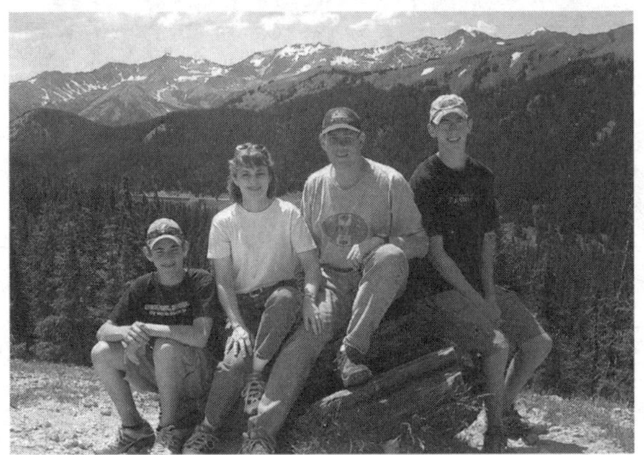

Wind River Ranch excursion to the Rocky Mountains, July 2005

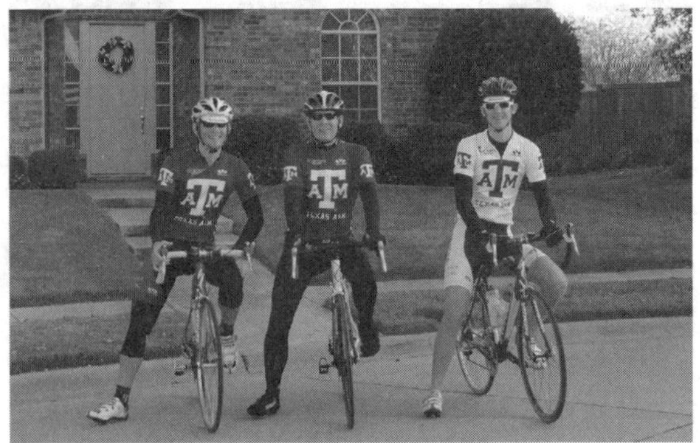

Shane and Chad with Chris, November 2009

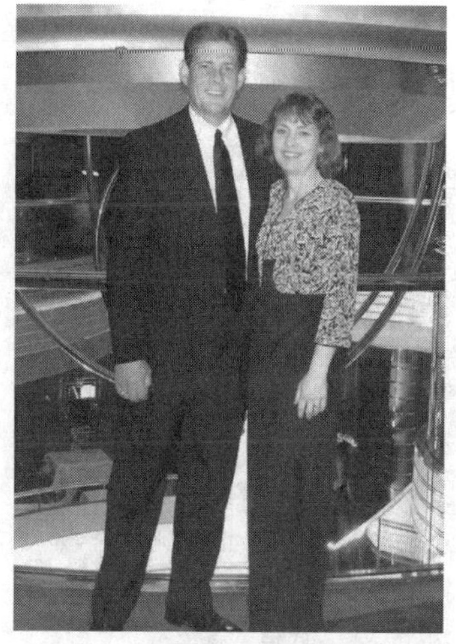

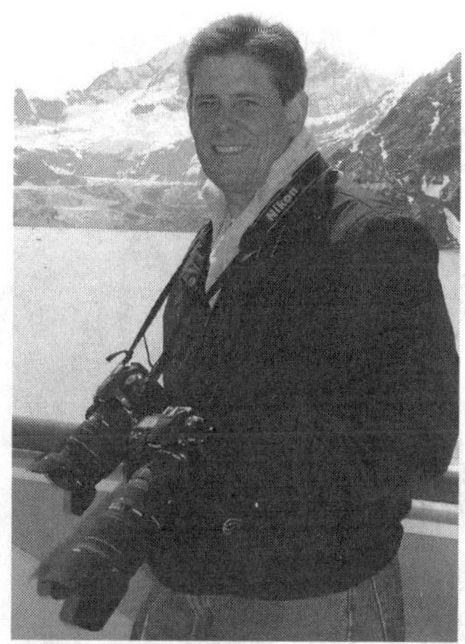

Celebrating our 25th wedding anniversary on a cruise to Alaska with Insight for Living, July 2009

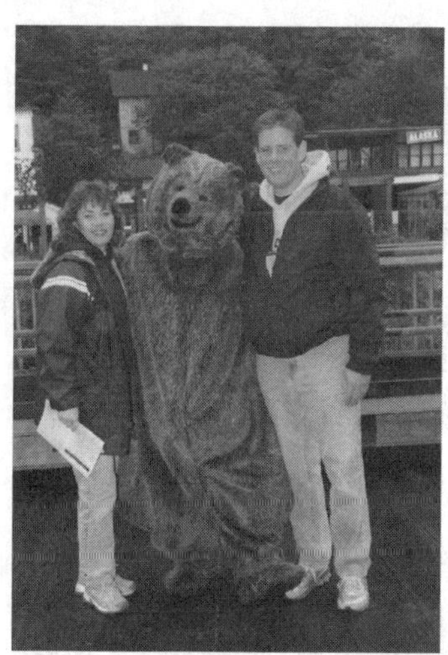

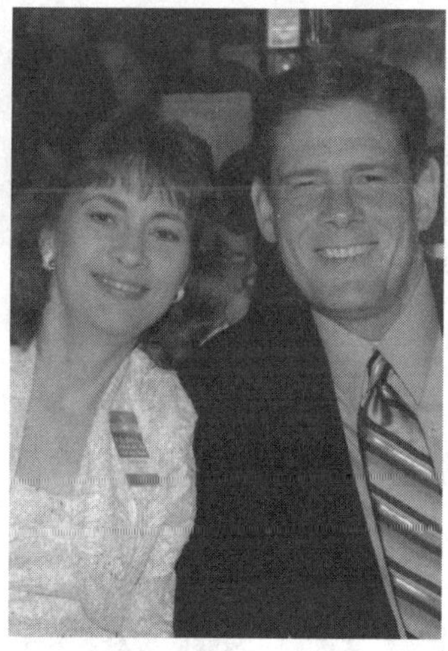

(Left) Juneau, Alaska
(Right) Formal dinner night

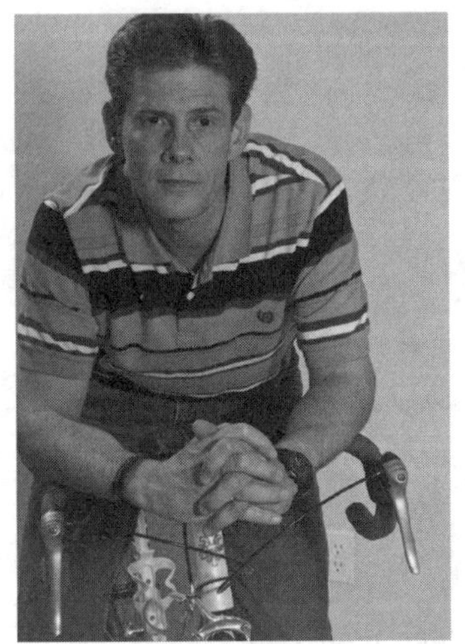

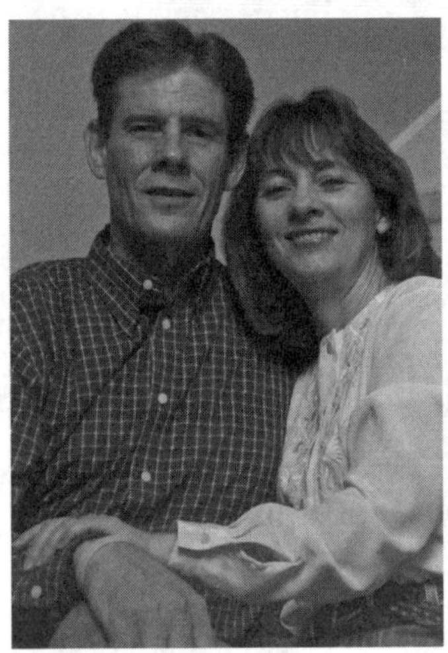

(Left) The day Chris was diagnosed with cancer, July 30, 2010
(Right) Three days before brain radiation, September 13, 2010

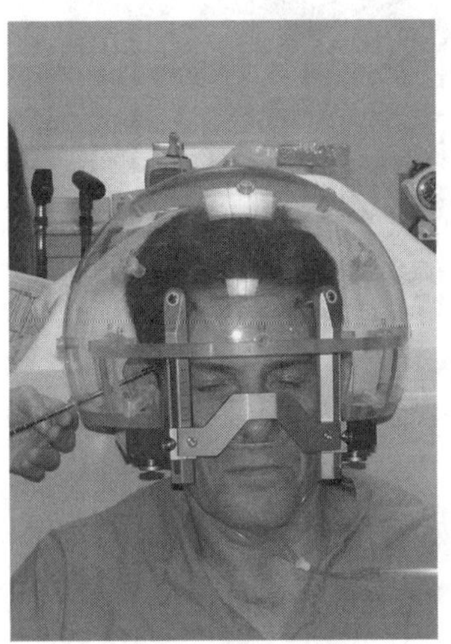

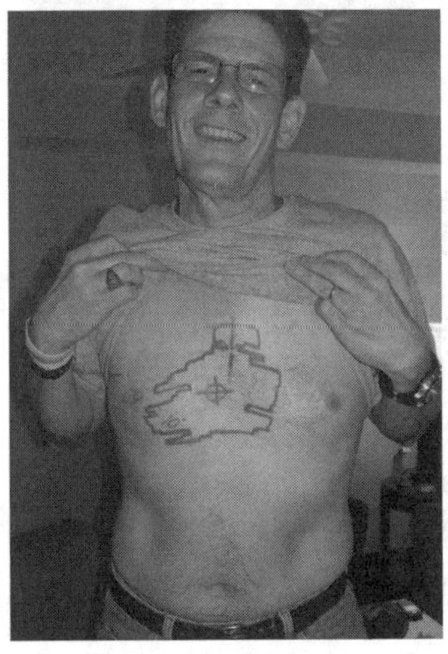

(Left) Getting measured for Gamma Knife, September 16, 2010
(Right) Target for radiation, October 27, 2010

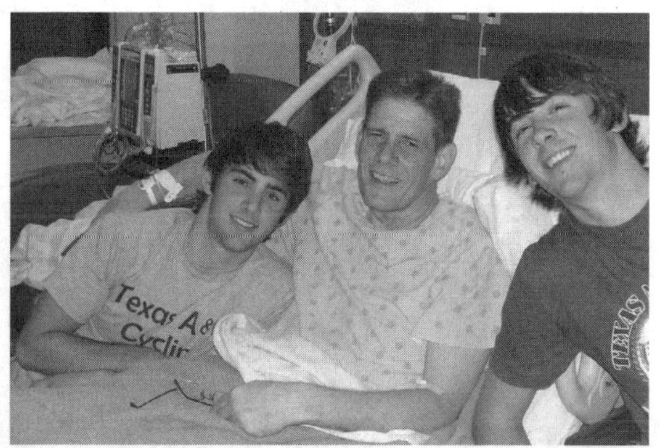

Shane and Chad providing hospital cheer, October 23, 2010

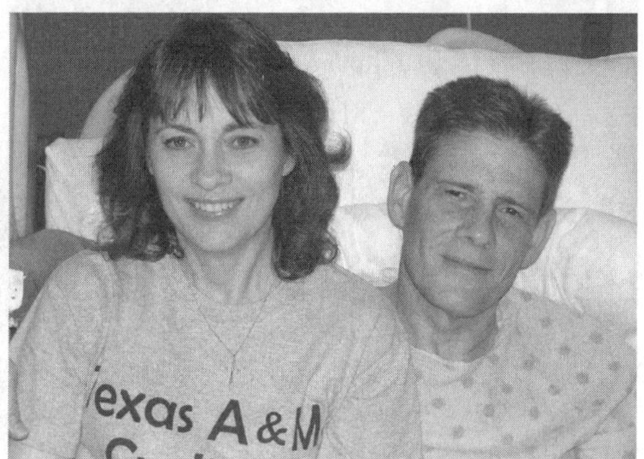

Chris attempting to smile with pneumonia—
again, October 23, 2010

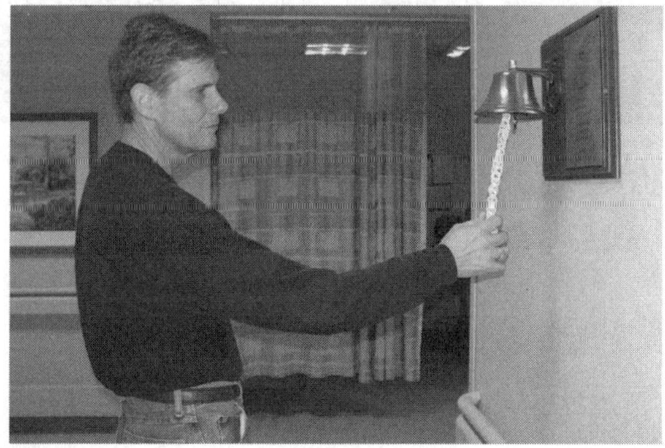

Celebrating the end of radiation, November 16, 2010

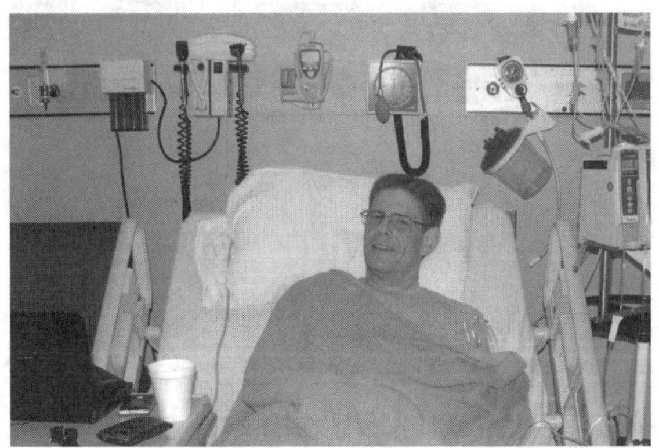

First chemo treatment, December 16, 2010

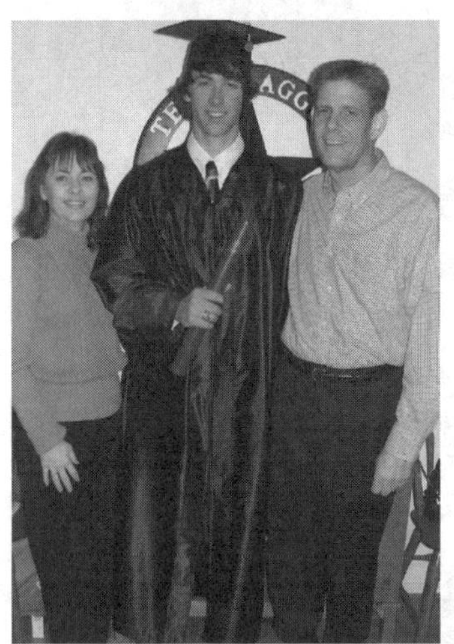

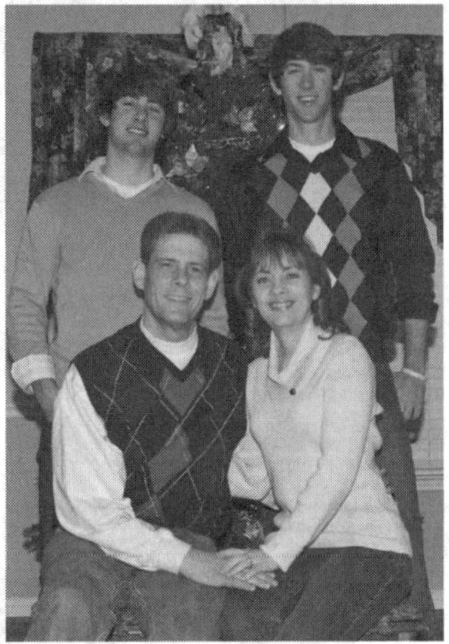

(Left) Chad's college graduation, December 17, 2010
(Right) Christmas day, 2010

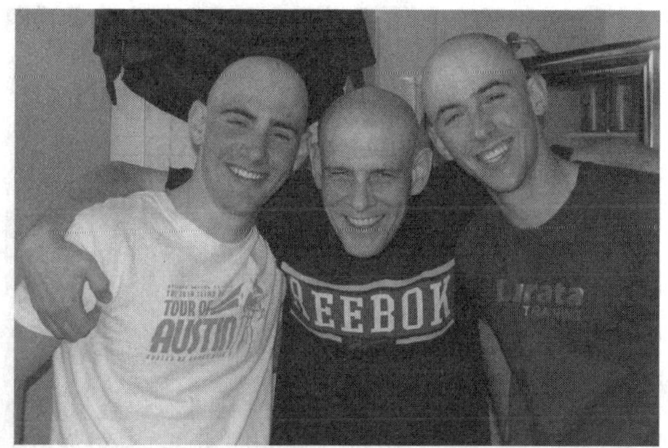

Three bald amigos, December 27, 2010

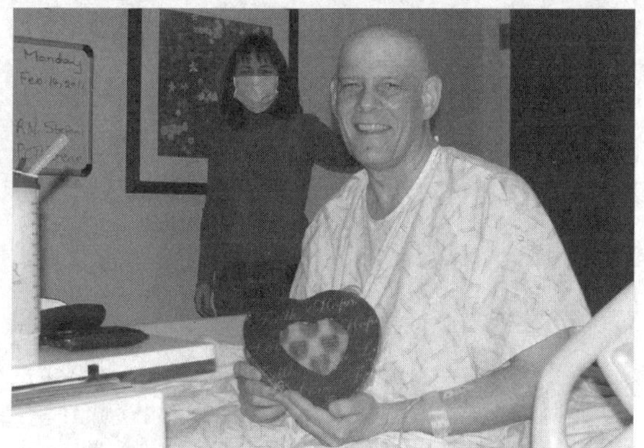

Hospitalized with neutropenia, Valentine's Day, 2011

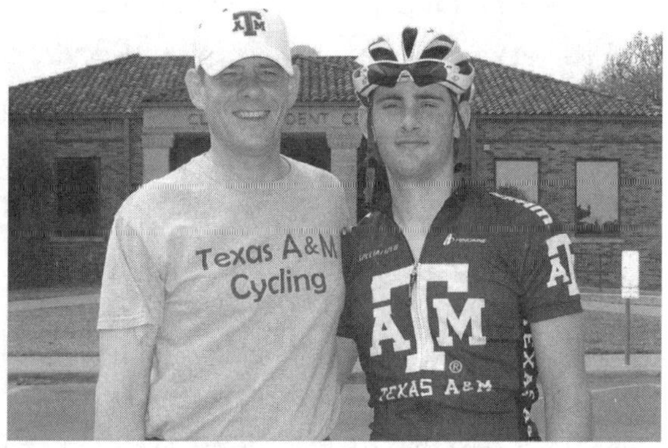

Surprised Shane at collegiate bike race, April 2011

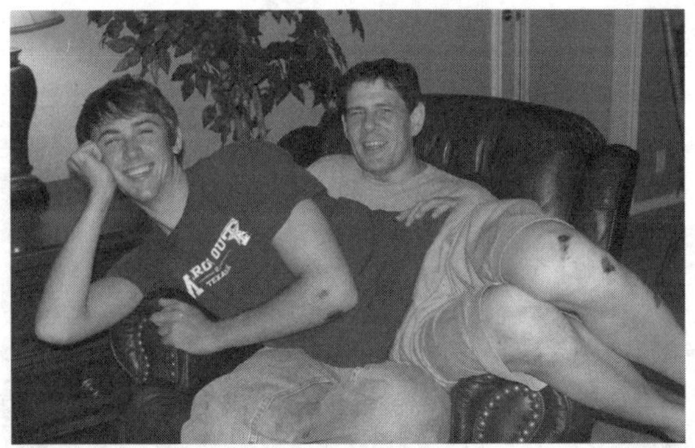

Chad was never too big for Pappy's lap, September 2011

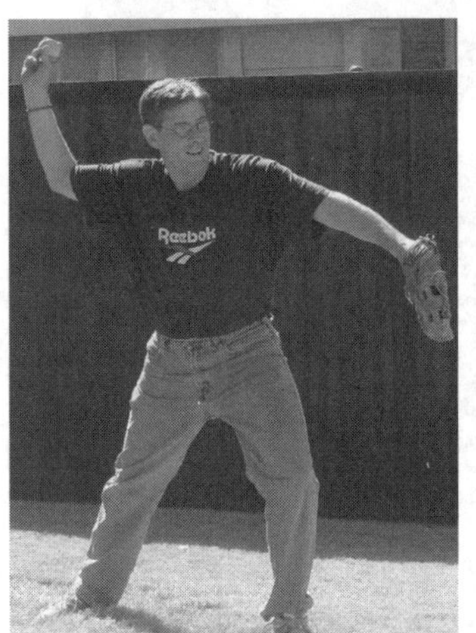

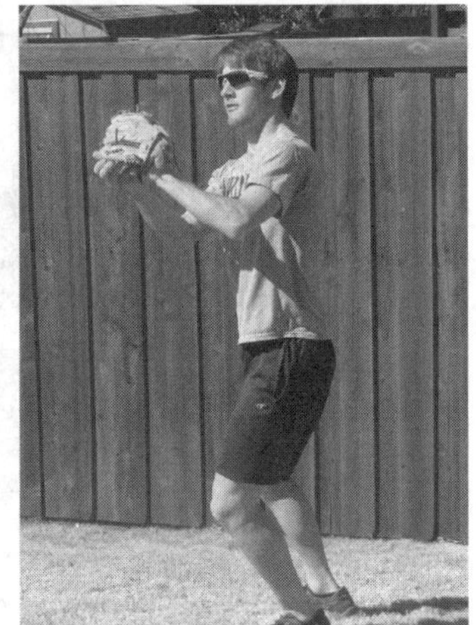

Playing catch with Shane, March 2013

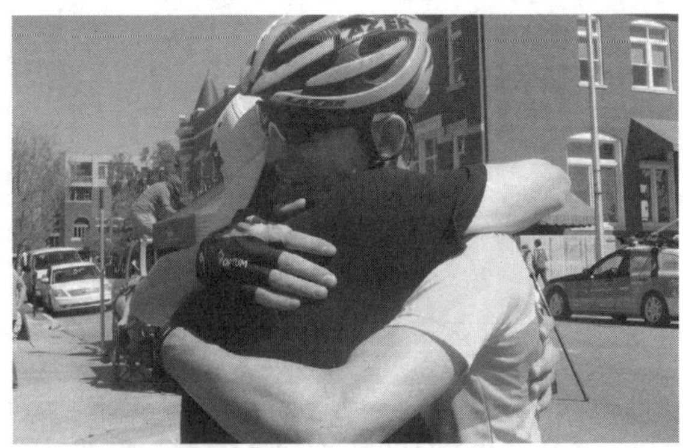

Dreams intersecting in Fayetteville, Arkansas, April 2013

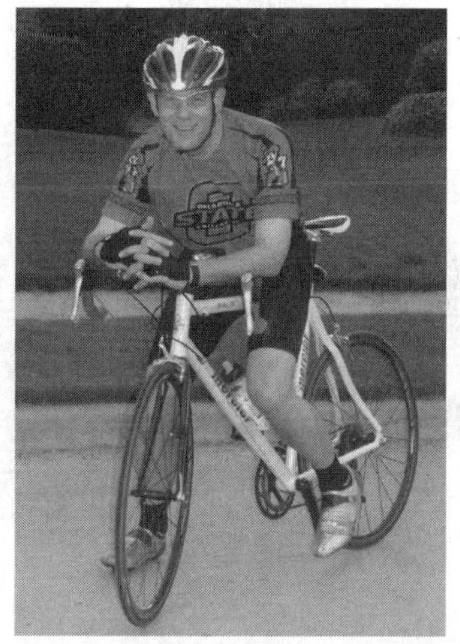

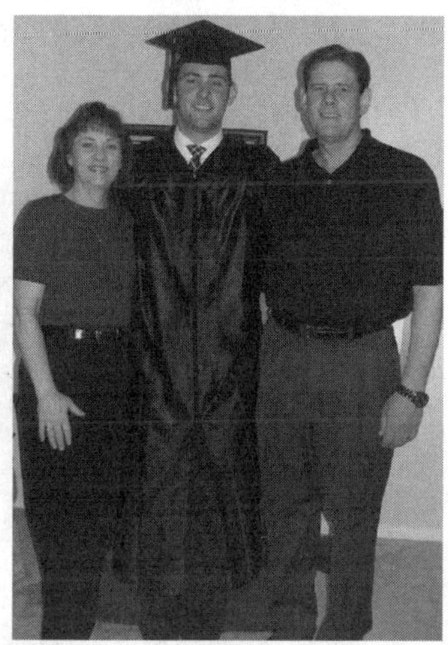

(Left) Saturday morning ride, June 2013
(Right) Shane's college graduation, August 16, 2013

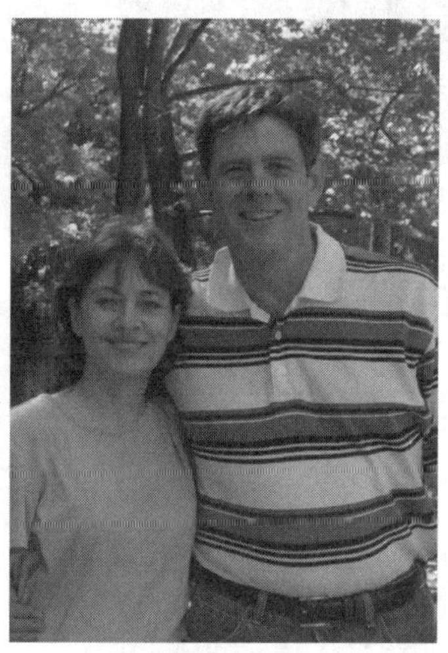

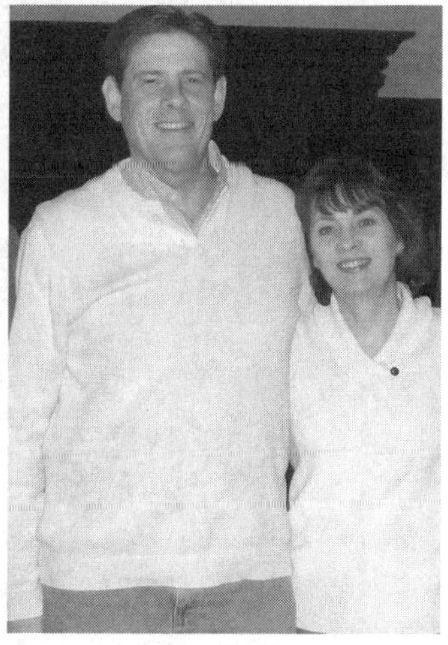

(Left) Dogwood Canyon Nature Park, October 2013
(Right) Thanksgiving 2013

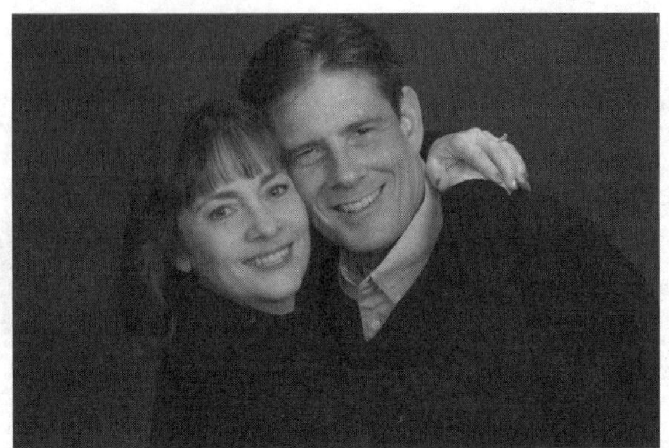

Married 30 years, 2014

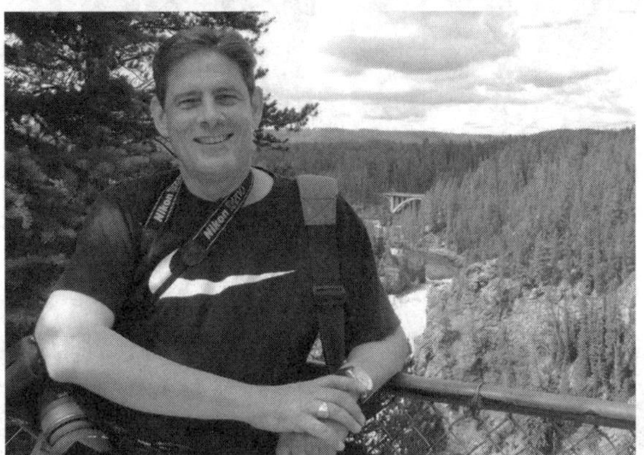

Yellowstone National Park, July 2015

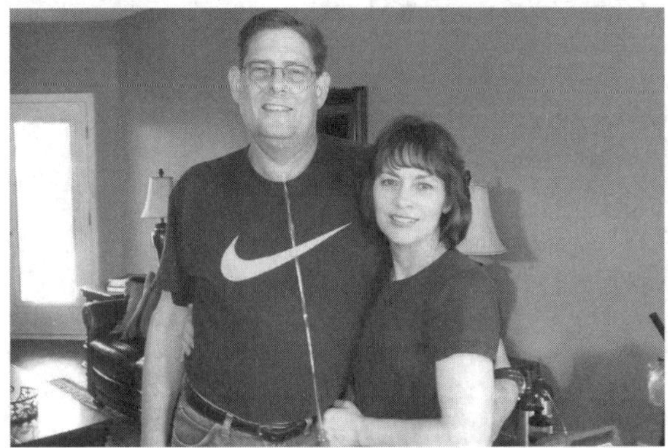

Chris on oxygen. Our last photo taken together, June 5, 2016

Chapter 21

FEVERS OF UNKNOWN ORIGIN

More MRI and CT scans were performed on September 11 per the trial protocol. By that evening, Chris had a fever. The "fevers of unknown origin" had become so predicable that, at the first warning signs and with the doctor's permission, Chris would take acetaminophen and an antibiotic before the fevers got out of control.

The doctors were so busy treating other patients that they didn't notice a pattern. Taking matters into my own hands, I turned to my three-ring binder, which meticulously chronicled Chris's treatments and health status. I sometimes wondered if the medical staff silently laughed at me every time I whipped out my binder at our appointments and every time a nurse came in his hospital room. But I didn't care. It was my way of helping the love of my life beat cancer.

I charted how soon the fevers started after a scan or medical procedure: four times within eight to twenty-four hours after a CT scan given with contrast dye. Was it a coincidence?

I searched online to see if contrast dye can cause a fever. It was listed as a possible side effect.

At our appointment that morning, I showed Dr. Schaefer my spreadsheet showing the correlation between the fevers and scans. As I suspected, he confirmed, "LDK378 is hard on the kidneys, and so is CT contrast. Maybe the combination of the medicine and the contrast is causing the problem, since blood tests haven't found any sign of infection."

He instructed Chris to take a low-dose steroid before the next scan to see if that would keep the fever at bay without having to take an antibiotic.

Whoever gives heed to instruction prospers, and blessed is he who trusts in the Lord.

—Proverbs 16:20 NIV

Chapter 22

IT'S A WONDERFUL LIFE

Back in 2010, Chris posted a blog entry titled "It's a Wonderful Life," referring to his favorite Christmas movie. He said the movie made him wonder, *Would it matter to anyone if I were not here? Have I made a difference to anyone?*

Prone to winter illness, Chris was frustrated easily and discouraged by a simple cold or fever. I gathered stories from people who had been a part of his life clear back to his childhood and put them in a notebook to surprise him on his birthday in November 2013. I asked them to share a funny or fond memory, something they admired or appreciated about him, something he had said or done to inspire them, or how he had influenced their life.

Chris became teary-eyed when he opened the notebook. He took it to another room to read it in private. I could hear him crying and blowing his nose, so I know it touched him deeply.

Here's a portion of what I wrote to Chris.

I'm amazed sometimes at your mental strength and determination to overcome obstacles in life, as well as your physical strength to push on when you don't feel like doing so. You've taught me that setbacks are only temporary. We must have faith to carry us through and let others carry us when we are too weary to continue on alone. I've learned that we are never really alone, though. When we aren't being lifted up by friends, family, and unknown angels, the Lord is carrying us over the hurdles of life.

I have gained so much from what we have gone through together, and although I always felt our marriage was strong, this journey has brought us even closer. I have learned so much from watching you battle "the beast." You have been a positive influence on my life and have shown me how to have faith even when things look hopeless. You have lived your faith.

I am so proud to see you jumping at every opportunity to provide encouragement to others with cancer, as others have encouraged us.

I feel honored and privileged to be able to witness one of God's miracles up close and personal. I am closer to God because I am so close to you.

"I came that they may have life, and have it abundantly."
—John 10:10

Chapter 23

BRAIN MYSTERY AND KIDNEY TOXICITY

In January 2014, after being in the clinical trial for a year, Chris was one of the few patients still able to tolerate LDK378 at full dosage. Most patients had too many complications and had to reduce their dose.

Two months earlier, Chris had felt bad for a week after taking steroids as instructed before scans, so he asked for a saline infusion instead to quickly flush the CT contrast dye from his kidneys. That didn't entirely prevent a fever, but it helped. Roughly eight hours after the CT scan, his temperature rose. Fortunately, he needed only acetaminophen and an ice pack to control the fever. Four hours later, he was back to normal.

Dr. Schaefer thought the fevers were being caused by the contrast dye and asked me to find out what type of contrast MD Anderson used since Chris never ran a fever after getting a CT scan there. I found out they used Omnipaque 350 contrast dye. Highlands Oncology Group used Optiray 300. Since Chris didn't have trouble with the Omnipaque contrast, they ordered it for him in Fayetteville. When Chris went for the CT scan in February, he received the Omnipaque contrast along with a saline infusion afterward. After battling the fevers for a year, we had found the right combination of treatments to successfully prevent them.

Four months later, Highlands Oncology Group switched all their patients to Omnipaque contrast and found they had fewer side effects. Patients were continuing to reap benefits from Chris's experience.

God confirmed we were seeking treatment at the right place, with a medical team that was willing to experiment with different methods to help him. We also found out UT Southwestern was referring their lung cancer patients to the clinic in Arkansas for the LDK378 study because the trial they thought would be opened in Dallas twelve months previously was still not approved. We were glad we didn't wait.

With the fever problem solved, what was next?

BRAIN MYSTERY

We found out the next concern the following day. The brain MRI showed a new area the doctors couldn't explain. The radiologist didn't think it was a tumor. It looked like something normally seen in a stroke patient, but Chris didn't have any stroke symptoms.

A neuroradiologist at Highlands Oncology Group reviewed Chris's MRI brain scans back to 2010. I had provided copies of all his records, including CDs of scans, and the area of concern was on scans as early as 2011.

"This might represent a low-grade primary brain cancer, but it would be impossible to biopsy. It could also be a ministroke," she said, recommending a magnetic resonance angiogram (MRA). They also performed an ultrasound of his carotid arteries to see if a blockage had caused a stroke. They found no blockage.

Our oncologists from Arkansas and Texas consulted each other and thought it could be a low-grade cancer that might not present itself for another two to three years. Even if it were biopsied, it probably wouldn't show disease.

When we requested a second opinion from the neuroradiologist at UT Southwestern, we were informed our insurance probably wouldn't pay for a second opinion to read scans done at another institution. After praying about it, we cancelled the request for the second opinion and chose to not pursue the brain matter (pun intended).

KIDNEY TOXICITY

In March, Chris's creatinine level on his blood test was at a toxic level for his kidneys, and he had to stop taking LDK378 for seven days. For the first time in four years since his diagnosis, he wasn't taking any medication to fight cancer or the side effects of chemo. He wasn't on any pain medications, antibiotics for pneumonia or fever, or medication to help with nausea or intestinal issues, and he wasn't on any blood thinners to prevent clots.

How did he celebrate? He indulged in grapefruit, a forbidden fruit while in treatment.

We were approaching the four-year mark of when Chris's symptoms first appeared. Being told there was something unexplainable in his scans was a reminder we had been on this odyssey longer than most. We were stepping into territory unfamiliar to us as well as to most doctors treating lung cancer.

> *Trust in the Lord with all your heart and do not lean on your own understanding. In all your ways acknowledge Him, and He will make your paths straight.*
>
> —Proverbs 3:5

Chapter 24

SNAKES AND DRINKING POISON

We attended a local concert where Christian artist Carman Licciardello was singing. Diagnosed with cancer in 2013, Carman was told to get his affairs in order and prepare to die. But a year after treatment and being declared disease-free, he was touring again.

After one of his songs, he asked his audience to stand up and join him in singing it again with him. Neither Chris nor I could open our mouths; we were choked up after hearing words we felt were meant for us. Wrapping our arms around each other's waist, tears streamed down our cheeks as everyone around us sang "Prayer." The song was about how nothing is impossible for those who faithfully believe. With prayer, the Lord can move a mountain and create miracles over and over again.

During the concert, Carman referenced an unfamiliar Scripture verse in the book of Mark. I made a mental note to look it up when we got home.

He asked those who needed healing to stand up and those surrounding to lay hands on them and pray for healing. I placed my hand on Chris's shoulder as Carman sang. I'm sure my makeup was all washed off after he finished singing "Jesus Heal Me."

As we drove in our driveway after the concert, the headlights shone on something in front of the garage door.

"What's that?" I asked.

It slithered across the entrance to the garage door.

As I totally freaked out, Chris ran around to the front door to get into the garage for a garden tool. He came back around to the driveway with a flashlight and a rake with hard steel tines. I courageously stood inside the truck with the door open and shined the flashlight on the snake while he beat it with the solid back side of the rake. It was one tough snake and kept slithering away. Chris corralled it with the rake tines and brought it back on the driveway where our flood lights gave extra visibility. He finally smashed its head, although the body kept twitching.

"It's dead enough. It can't bite anyone," he said.

I opened the garage door and got a garbage bag. He picked up the snake with the rake and dropped it in. I felt brave enough the next day to open the trash bin to see if it had escaped. By the smell of things, I think it was truly dead enough.

Was this snake incident a coincidence? That was the first snake we had seen on our property in the sixteen years we had lived there. What are the odds that of all the places the snake could have been, it was in the only place we would have seen it that night?

I got my reminder to look up that Scripture verse. And I sensed God was telling us the chemo would continue to heal Chris.

> *"They will pick up snakes with their hands; and when they drink deadly poison, it will not hurt them at all; they will place their hands on sick people, and they will get well."*
>
> —MARK 16:18 NIV

Chapter 25

NOT TAKING NED FOR GRANTED

April 29, 2014, was another historic day in the lung cancer world. LDK378 was FDA approved via the fast track. The brand name for this drug became Zykadia. According to a media release, Zykadia was one of the first medicines to be approved following FDA Breakthrough Therapy designation due to the significance of results observed in the trial and the serious and life-threatening nature of ALK-positive non-small cell lung cancer. In 2017, it was FDA approved as a first-line treatment for patients like Chris.

Of all the patients in the phase II clinical trials, two had a complete response when it was approved. That might not sound like much, but for someone with stage IV lung cancer, that is a miracle. It was enough to convince the FDA to approve the drug. Again, I like to think Chris was one of the two miracles since he was the first patient in the U.S. in the phase II trials.

He was doing great in June. We rode bikes together in the neighborhood. One evening, he suddenly felt ornery and sped off ahead, leaving me in his dust. It took me almost two blocks to catch up, proving he still had spunk left in his lungs. I don't know who was more elated—me or Chris.

Although he had twice defeated stage IV lung cancer and was feeling well, I wasn't taking "no evidence of disease" for granted. I knew there was no guarantee the disease wouldn't return, and the odds weren't in his favor. It was likely just a matter of time.

Chris had been taking LDK378 for more than sixteen months. The average length of response for patients was only seven months. I began to feel moments of panic because we didn't have a backup plan. It takes time to find and process treatment options. With lung cancer, we didn't always have the luxury of time. With my woman's intuition giving me a sense of urgency, I started investigating new studies on June 17. After several hours in the business center at the Fayetteville hotel before our appointment, I printed data on clinical trials and research study results I had found. My head was spinning with information overload.

When I discussed the trials with Dr. Schaefer later that day, he said some of the drugs were so new he hadn't heard of them yet. He smiled at Chris and said, "I don't think we'll need to change treatment plans anytime soon. In fact, I'm so pleased with the way you're responding to treatment, I've scheduled your future appointments through the end of the year. I feel you'll be on this chemo for a long time."

People occasionally asked us how long Chris would be in treatment. They didn't realize that patients with advanced lung cancer almost always need to be in continuous treatment for the rest of their lives. Chris was taking a drug that inhibits the growth of cancer containing the ALK gene. The disease comes back because it finds a way around the medication, similar to the way bacteria becomes resistant to antibiotics. He would be on a specific treatment as long as it worked.

I went a month without writing in my daily journal. No news was good news, and there was nothing worth documenting. That was about to change.

At our appointment on July 14, Dr. Schaefer said Chris's lungs sounded clear, his edema had improved, and his labs still looked good. His fatigue and breathing exercises had improved. But despite all this good news, Chris began coughing a little.

The next evening at supper, his voice was a little hoarse when he said the blessing.

"That's not a good sign," he said. "I'm afraid the cancer is back."

Did he know his body that well, or was he just being paranoid? Truth be told, I had the same fear. That's what cancer does to the mind. Every little ache or symptom makes the mind leap to the conclusion that it's the disease. Four years prior, he had attributed the same symptoms to allergies. He was trying to not be apprehensive, but his cough worsened.

Be on your guard; stand firm in the faith; be men of courage; be strong.

—1 CORINTHIANS 16:13 NIV

Chapter 26

HEADING INTO UNKNOWN LAND

By July 29, 2014, Chris was coughing a little more and said he felt like he was breathing through a straw. A week later, his cough was harder and more frequent, and the hoarseness was worse. He was only pulling 3,000 on the incentive spirometer. One evening while resting my head on his chest, I could hear a sticky clicking in his lungs. I hadn't heard that ominous sound in a long time. We fully suspected the cancer had returned.

We soon discovered that our instincts were right.

The CT scan on August 12 showed a spot in Chris's right lung was enlarging. The chemo was still working, just not at 100 percent capacity. Even though we had tried to prepare ourselves, it was difficult to hear the news as the doctor showed us the scan on the computer monitor. I thought my heart would pound out of my chest.

Because of disease progression, Chris had to leave the clinical trial. Novartis allowed him to continue the trial medication at no cost to us for "compassionate use" until he found another viable treatment.

Dr. Schaefer recommended targeted therapy, immunotherapy, or standard chemo. The first two choices, unfortunately, weren't available in Fayetteville. We had become fond of our medical team, and saying good-bye to them was tough. It took all my strength to fight off tears when hugging Dr. Schaefer good-bye.

Continuing to research clinical trials, I called a biopharmaceutical company about a new drug in Tennessee. They were opening a phase I trial for RXDX-101 in Houston in mid-August.

Chris and I called Dr. Heymach at MD Anderson and discussed six clinical trial options. The doctor also suggested Alimta. Cancer cells tend to forget what standard chemo looks like, so Chris could do chemo for a couple of rounds to kill the cells that weren't yet resistant to chemo.

I left a phone message for the principal investigator of a clinical trial at the University of Colorado. He's nationally known in the lung cancer world and does seminars to educate patients and doctors.

Amazingly, he took the time to personally call me back that evening and recommended four options. He agreed the standard chemo was a good alternative since Chris had only one round of it, adding, "The cancer may be resistant to the targeted therapy but not recognize Alimta."

Dr. Gerber at UT Southwestern recommended a clinical trial for AT13387.

Chris admitted on CaringBridge that he was discouraged:

I realize I was naive when first diagnosed, thinking I'd kick cancer's tail and move on. The second diagnosis rattled me, but, again, I thought I'd just change medicines and continue with life. This third diagnosis is a real kick in the gut. This is the first time I have doubts about beating the beast in my chest. We're not ignorant about the odds that I now face in beating this, but those are man's stats, not God's plan. Even though there is doubt, disbelief, and discouragement, we still have hope.

We held on to the conviction that God specializes in the impossible. Unlike the first recurrence, though, there was no real clear-cut, obvious next line of attack. Even the doctors didn't agree on what to recommend next since this was new territory for them. We didn't enjoy being at the forefront of lung cancer treatment advances, but we had no choice.

Several drugs were being tested, but Chris would not qualify for those studies. Most trials were restricted to those who had taken no inhibitor drugs or no more than one. We wanted to avoid phase I or phase III trials since we'd determined that phase II offered the best chance. Most of the studies were out of state, requiring a lot of driving time or flying.

Facing a decision based on the unknown was scary. We had to decide on a drug for which solid results existed for only a few patients. Some trials were so new, the oncologists hadn't heard of them, or the study results weren't published yet. We didn't want to waste valuable time on drugs that might not help, but God hadn't answered our prayers yet for discernment.

We were thinking we might have to resort to "Eeny, meeny, miny, moe" when Chris wrote "Unknown Land."

The Sunday morning we were packing for our last trip to Fayetteville, the words God spoke to Abram popped into my head. God told Abram to pack all his belongings and move to a "land that I will show you." Those words have been stuck in my head as we've been evaluating the different drug trials that are available. We've been seeking God's direction to find the best plan for me. While we've narrowed down the choices to two or three drugs, there still doesn't appear to be a clear path. We're heading into unknown land.

The one thing we do know is that God will show us the land we're to go to, and He will be waiting for us when we arrive.

Let me hear Your lovingkindness in the morning; for I trust in You; teach me the way in which I should walk; for to You I lift up my soul.

—Psalm 143:8

Chapter 27

THIRD CLINICAL TRIAL

God was finally directing our path for the next treatment. I found out the first three human patients had been enrolled in phase I for RXDX-101 at a very low dose. They wouldn't open enrollment for the next group for another four weeks. This trial didn't look like a wise choice.

MD Anderson had expanded the phase I study for X-396 to include patients who had been on more than one inhibitor drug, so Chris could get in. It had completed the dose-escalation phase, and he could enroll immediately at the maximum tolerated dose. We decided to go for it.

Chris had a PET scan in Houston on August 27, 2014, which confirmed disease in his right lung. A new growth was pinching off an airway, causing him to cough more.

We met with Dr. Davis and Justina, the research nurse. We discovered we had three hurdles:

1. The drug manufacturer, Xcovery, required a biopsy.
2. Chris's creatinine level was 1.51, and the study required it to be less than 1.5.

3. The radiologist had to classify what was seen on the PET as being "measurable progression of disease." If it couldn't be measured, he couldn't be in the clinical trial.

We left Houston on August 29, not expecting to go back for a couple of weeks since it was Labor Day weekend, and scheduling appointments would be difficult. Thirty minutes after we got home, we received a call from MD Anderson. They wanted Chris to start the study the following Friday.

HOPE AND FAITH

Although we hadn't received final word that Chris could start the new drug, we headed for Houston the next week on blind faith that God would coordinate everything in His perfect timing. Based on our past experiences, we had hope that God would fulfill His promises to take care of us, even before those promises materialized.

> *But hope that is seen is no hope at all. Who hopes for what he already has? But if we hope for what we do not yet have, we wait for it patiently.*
>
> —Romans 8:24–25 NIV

Fortunately, we didn't have to wait patiently for long. As soon as we pulled out of the driveway, Chris's cell phone rang. Justina was calling to tell us the radiologist had classified the growth as measurable. While still on the phone with her, Chris received a voice message that the biopsy had been scheduled. We headed for Houston, confident he would be starting X-396 on Friday. We couldn't help but smile at God's timing in response to our faith.

> *Now faith is the assurance of things hoped for, the conviction of things not seen. . . . And without faith it is impossible to*

> *please Him, for he who comes to God must believe that He is and that He is a rewarder of those who seek Him.*
>
> —HEBREWS 11:1, 6

BASELINE TESTS

Chris had blood tests, three EKGs five minutes apart, and a prebiopsy appointment on September 3. The next day, he had a baseline eye test for the study. His creatinine level was worse and was up to 1.53. However, the study allowed for a higher level if his creatinine clearance ratio was okay. They had calculated that, and Xcovery agreed he could get in the trial. We had one last appointment with the oncologist to get his approval to proceed. Then it was off to get a lung biopsy.

Anne and Warner, our research nurses during the crizotinib clinical trial, heard we were in the building. They came to see us, but Chris was getting the biopsy done. We had grown fond of these two nurses. It made our day to know they came to see us on their lunch break. I got to chat with them for ten minutes and snapped a photo to show Chris.

For those who feel they would be "just a number" at a large cancer center, this shows that the medical team truly cares about the patients and caregivers as individuals.

PHASE I TRIAL, DAY 1

We checked in at 8:00 a.m. on September 5 at the special clinic where phase I trials were conducted. Chris was supposed to have his first dose around 9:00. He wasn't allowed to eat within two hours before or after taking the drug, so he made sure breakfast was finished by 7:00.

At 10:30, Justina came in—not a good sign.

"Xcovery is withholding approval because your ALK gene mutation analysis report is four years old," she said. "I've been in a battle with them all morning because the study wasn't written to require a new analysis. All the tissue from yesterday's biopsy has been sent to them for experimental use. We weren't allowed to keep any tissue since they are paying for the biopsy. Do you want to reschedule starting the drug or wait another ninety minutes to see if I can convince them to accept the four-year-old report?"

The testing was an all-day event, and we were partly into the day. A line had already been placed in his arm for the hourly blood tests—after much difficulty.

"I don't want to go through that again," Chris answered. "I'll wait."

Thankfully, we were blessed with a coordinator who went to battle for Chris. She continued to call and fight. Just before noon, we got approval to proceed.

We quickly learned that a phase I trial is a lot more involved than a phase II trial. Extra precautions ensure the drug is not dangerously toxic to humans since it's the start of human testing. They continually monitor with tests. During the next eight hours, he had eighteen EKGs and eight blood draws at scheduled intervals to see how his body handled the drug and to make sure he didn't have serious adverse reactions. He was finally dismissed at 8:30 p.m.

Being cooped up in a tiny hospital room with his medical team going in and out all day took a toll on him. Since this is a teaching hospital, they came in teams of two, with the students sometimes doing the procedure. The EKG machine and nurse's carts filled up the space not occupied by the medical professionals. Even I felt claustrophobic.

Chris was physically and mentally exhausted after the long, stressful day. When we got back to the hotel, all he could do was sit on the couch and stare at the wall. He didn't even turn on the TV. It was almost an hour before he could move to get ready for bed.

He had to be back at the clinic the next afternoon for another blood draw twenty-four hours after the first dose, and then we headed for home.

ORANGES

A week later, we arrived for an early blood draw per the trial protocol but learned Chris had to see the oncologist first for approval. We tried to reschedule our 2:00 appointment to that morning, but Dr. Davis was booked solid. They said they would try to work Chris in. I guess we were spoiled. We had been told clinical trial patients get priority treatment because of the time-sensitive nature of trial protocol. That seemed to ring true in the past. But not that day. Five frustrating hours later, we got to see the doctor.

"How are you feeling?" he asked.

"I'm not coughing as often or as hard," Chris said.

"That's better than a CT scan." He authorized Chris to continue on X-396 and left the exam room less than five minutes later. Then it was off to get the blood test.

Chris hadn't eaten since early morning. The longer things stretched on, the hungrier he got, and the more his frustration grew. He finally took the pills around 2:00, and we were allowed to leave the clinic. He couldn't get out fast enough and practically ran to the truck. He wanted nothing to do with Houston and asked me to drive. Although he'd never had road rage, I think he might have succumbed to it that day if he were driving.

He still couldn't eat for another two hours and was ravenous when we got to Huntsville at 4:00. Chris wanted pancakes, so we found a local IHOP restaurant.

The irritations of the day and seeing Chris like this brought me down fast. Tears blurred my eyes, and I could hardly read the menu. After the waiter took our order, Chris laid his head in his hands and closed his eyes. I escaped to the bathroom to have a good cry. I returned to our table as Roy, our teenaged waiter, approached. Chris was still resting with his eyes closed.

Seeing the bandage on my husband's arm, Roy assumed he had donated blood. "Would you like some orange juice for a little pick-me-up?" Roy asked. "No charge."

"No thanks on the juice," Chris replied, "but if you could find an orange, I would really appreciate it." Orange juice caused Chris to have acid reflux, but he could usually eat oranges. Having never seen them on the menu, I thought he had just asked for the impossible. I wept again, but this time, with gratitude. Roy's unexpected kindness pulled my heartstrings.

"I don't think we have oranges, but I'll go check."

"No way he brings back an orange. If he does, it'll be a small miracle," Chris said, his voice cracking with emotion.

Just a few minutes later, Roy returned with a small bowl of canned oranges. "We just got these in for some reason," he said, then apologized for not having fresh fruit.

Chris and I teared up. God had sent us a caring waiter to nourish both body and soul with canned oranges—something normally not in stock at that restaurant. I felt like God was saying, *Remember, I delight in delivering even small miracles. Here ya go.*

We were so appreciative, Chris asked to speak with the manager. Roy thought he was about to get in trouble, but he got the manager anyway.

"We had a long, frustrating day at a cancer center," Chris explained. "When Roy saw I was having a rough day, he went beyond the call of duty to make me feel better. Most young men wouldn't have been so thoughtful. I wanted to make sure you knew you have a great employee."

We left a generous tip, and on the way out, Chris spoke with Roy. He expressed our appreciation and told him he had put in a good word with the manager. He hugged the waiter and then walked to the truck. This time there was a little spring in his step.

Chris later recalled this incident in "A Collection of Randomness."

> *It wasn't about the oranges. It was that someone saw we weren't having a good day and took a few moments to care. Sometimes you may see someone in need and think that what you have to offer won't make a difference and move on. That small gesture may not mean much to you, but it may be the high point of that person's day.*

If Chris and I had felt God's love only when He healed my husband, then we would have missed the small thrills in life that He brought—such as canned oranges. We learned to look for moments of joy in the midst of our trials, and we found them, experiencing God as never before.

God is always close by. It's up to us to find Him. Sometimes it's obvious His hand is at work. Other times it's easy to miss, such as the prompting of a friend calling when we need someone to talk to. This is one of the Lord's ways of showing us we aren't alone and He cares.

BAD RASH

On the eighth day of taking X-396, things went downhill. Chris ran a low-grade fever, and red blotches appeared on his face. His face was in extreme pain, and he kept cold wash cloths on it all day. He woke up during the night feeling like someone was holding a blow torch to his face. His face was as red as a lobster, and he had a full-blown rash and itchy scalp. We tried ointments, acetaminophen, and an antihistamine to get him some relief, but nothing helped. Putting wet frozen wash cloths on his face gave temporary relief, but the pain was intense, and the rash was spreading.

We called Justina on September 15 and sent her a photo of his red face. She told him to stop taking X-396 immediately and sent prescriptions for an antibiotic and face cream to our pharmacy. He was having a grade 2 side effect. Chris was disappointed to stop the drug after just ten days, even if only temporarily.

That afternoon, his eyelids and face got puffy, and the rash was spreading to his chest and shoulders. The next day, red spots spread to his arms, and his entire face swelled. He was so miserable he would occasionally scream in agony.

At one point he said, "This must be what hell is like—constant, burning torment and no relief."

It was difficult to watch him suffer, unable to relieve the torture.

We were back in Houston the afternoon of September 17. The drug had caused his skin to feel bumpy, like the skin of an orange. I dropped him off and parked near MD Anderson to wait. We didn't want to pay for parking when he would be there only for a lab draw.

When I picked him up, he broke into tears as soon as he got in the car. "It took the lab technician two tries to draw blood."

That wasn't unusual.

"I'm tired of being in pain," he sobbed.

I was concerned. *If he's this miserable now, what's it going to be like if things get worse? He's had it relatively easy compared to other lung cancer patients we've known.*

We went out for supper, and while waiting for our food, he was in distress from the face rash. I ran and got ice cubes in paper towels for him to put on his face. We ignored strange glances.

At his follow-up appointment the next day, Dr. Davis and Justina realized the rash was much worse than they had thought. Chris was told to stay off the drug for another week. The study required he not be off the medicine more than fourteen days. He was given more ammunition to combat the side effects.

We received good news that his creatinine was back in an acceptable range. Having his blood drawn late in the day gave him a chance to hydrate and improve his number, so we decided to continue that regimen instead of the early-morning lab draws.

Within the first day on the antibiotic, steroid, and topical prescriptions, Chris's face greatly improved and continued improving rapidly throughout the week. He was allowed to restart X-396 after being off eleven days. The protocol was a repeat of day one with eight hours of EKGs and blood draws, except without all the drama.

By September 27, his face looked nice, smooth, and soft like a baby's. He looked young again. Three days later, he started doing his breathing exercises again and was able to pull 3,000 on the incentive spirometer.

But by mid-October, Chris had a rash on his arms and back, his skin texture changed and was tender and itchy, and he was napping a lot. He was pulling only 2,500 on the incentive spirometer, when he was lucky. His lungs made strange noises when he breathed. And his coughing spells were so hard, I was afraid he'd pass out.

ANOINTING WITH OIL

Shane was leading a Bible study with his friends on the book of James. He called us on October 26 and said one part kept sticking out to him.

> *Is anyone among you sick? Then he must call for the elders of the church and they are to pray over him, anointing him with oil in the name of the Lord; and the prayer offered in faith will restore the one who is sick, and the Lord will raise him up, and if he has committed sins, they will be forgiven him.*
>
> —James 5:14–15 NIV

"I think Pappy qualifies as sick," Shane said. He suggested we ask our church elders to anoint his dad with oil.

I contacted our church that week. After the service on Sunday, we met with the elders. They asked Chris to tell them about his health situation. They were touched by his testimony of how God had been taking care of him and using his journey to reach others. Laying hands on Chris, they prayed over him and anointed him with oil. It was quite a moving experience. Even the elders, who had never met him before, were wiping away tears.

Although he wasn't miraculously healed at that moment, I immediately felt at peace with God's will.

KICKED OUT

We went back to Houston for his checkup on October 30. Chris's cough had improved again, he was feeling better, and his breathing exercises were improving. We thought he was turning a corner and expected the scans to show improvement.

We were blindsided when the cancer showed progression from the previous scans.

I felt the disease had flared when he was off the treatment and was improving once back on. But because the disease had progressed, Chris was kicked out of the X-396 clinical trial. We were back to square one again in finding a treatment.

BRAIN MATTER

The radiologist at MD Anderson was worried about the spot in Chris's brain that had been there for years. When comparing his MRI to one done in 2012, they observed a big change and noted the growth as "worrisome." This was a big deal, because most drug trials are written to preclude patients who have brain metastases until the brain mets are treated.

Chris consulted with a radiation oncologist and a neurosurgeon in Houston. They recommended doing nothing.

"The spot is near the center in the area that controls your motor movements. You passed all the motor tests during examination. Comparing the MRI to more recent ones from Arkansas, we're confident this is very slow growing and not related to the lung cancer. There's a slim possibility that it's some type of brain cancer, but we really don't believe that because you have no symptoms."

"What would we do if a study requires there be a negative diagnosis of a brain metastasis before I could start a new drug?" Chris asked.

"The first option would be to do an MR spectroscopy. This is a more specialized MRI that looks at metabolic activity to see if it's malignant. The results would probably be inconclusive."

The doctor continued, "The second option would be to perform a biopsy. We aren't in favor of this because of the location that would have to be biopsied. If you were to develop a clot or any bleeding post biopsy, there would be loss of some amount of motor skills. Because of the type of growth we're seeing, we aren't sure we could collect any tissue that would determine anything, because nothing lit up as cancerous. In other words, the risk isn't worth the potential reward. Gamma Knife isn't an option because the area is too big. We could do partial brain radiation, if necessary, but that would require thirty treatments over six weeks and would cause a delay in chemo."

We all agreed that since Chris had no symptoms of brain cancer, treating his lung cancer was the priority.

In his heart a man plans his course, but the Lord determines his steps.

—Proverbs 16:9 NIV

Chapter 28

LUNG CANCER AWARENESS AND PROGRESS

Our friend Cindy passed away from lung cancer at age thirty-nine, and we attended her funeral in Houston on November 1, 2014. That day was difficult for both of us. With Cindy's passing, four of the lung cancer patients we had become friends with and mentors to had died. They didn't live as long with the diagnosis as Chris had. He had a little bit of survivor's guilt because he was diagnosed first.

"Why am I still here and they're not?" he asked.

Cindy's death strengthened his determination to be a voice for people who can no longer speak for themselves here on earth. He wanted to raise awareness of this despicable disease and get it the attention it deserves.

The media has done a fantastic job of teaching our society that smoking can cause cancer. Now another harmful influence is causing deaths from lung cancer in those who have never smoked due to delayed diagnosis—stigma. People, including many doctors, still think that only smokers get the disease.

Invariably, when Chris told someone he had lung cancer, they would ask, "Did you smoke?" I became so frustrated with this that I started answering that question before it was asked.

We were mystified why the number one cause of cancer deaths could be one of the lowest funded and least talked about. People assume those with the disease brought it upon themselves. That's like saying to a woman with breast cancer, "It's your fault you have cancer because you have breasts." If you have lungs, you can get lung cancer.

We heard the same story *every* time we met new patients who had never smoked; they weren't diagnosed until they were already stage IV. Their doctors didn't suspect this disease because of their lack of smoking history. The disease is hard to treat if it's not caught early. By stage IV, there's a poor five-year survival rate.

The face of lung cancer is changing. Every year, more never-smokers are diagnosed. They're being diagnosed in their twenties and thirties—and even as young as age nine—with no typical symptoms. According to the American Cancer Society, more women die every year from lung cancer than from breast cancer.

Chris's early medical reports from when he was originally diagnosed documented, "The patient claims to have never smoked." This led me to believe they suspected he probably smoked at some point in his life, causing his own disease.

Although I was disappointed they didn't correctly diagnose Chris's condition, I was never angry. Instead, I decided to educate the medical professionals in our area about the stigma of lung cancer and its influence on misdiagnosis.

I sent a letter to several primary care physicians and pulmonologists in our hometown. I needed something good to come from Chris's bout with the disease. Below is an excerpt:

> *Lung cancer kills more people than breast, prostate, and colon cancer combined, but comes with the stigma that it could have been avoided by not smoking. However, 10%–20% of lung cancer patients (like my husband) have*

never smoked. Please help raise awareness among doctors and share this letter with them. If your patients have a cough that won't go away, please suggest a CT scan (not just an x-ray) more quickly if you can't diagnose a problem that could be related to lung cancer. Just because a person has never smoked doesn't mean they aren't at risk for this horrible disease. Early detection rarely happens in lung cancer patients—especially in never-smokers. You can help change this in the medical profession.

I included Chris's business card that contained his photo and a link to his blog. I also gave the doctors permission to contact me for more information about the disease in never-smokers, but no one ever did. Had I wasted my time? During one of my own doctor appointments, I handed Chris's business card to him. The doctor immediately realized this was the patient that another doctor in the building had told him about. Word was getting out after all.

Although there's never a good time to have cancer, this is an exciting era with scientific breakthroughs becoming increasingly common that extend the quality of life for survivors. I have hope that a cure for the disease will be found in the near future. Researchers continue to make great strides in understanding the biology behind cancer and developing new ways to deal with it. In June 2016, the FDA approved the use of liquid biopsies from blood samples to screen for certain mutations of lung cancer. This allows physicians to quickly identify the gene and determine individualized treatments known to work. This is less risky for the patient than lung biopsies. Some patients may be too sick to withstand a tissue biopsy, or the tumor may be located where obtaining a tissue sample wouldn't be safe. A collapsed lung is always a risk during a needle biopsy.

By participating in these groundbreaking studies, Chris helped advance science to fight the disease. For that, I am thankful, and so was he. There must be a special place in heaven for people who participate in clinical trials to help find a cure that will benefit others, risking their own health. Yes, the patients may benefit from the studies, but not always. The drug dosage could be too low or too high. They could have a toxic adverse reaction to the medication. Frequent monitoring is required through x-rays, brain MRIs, CT scans, and blood work. Radiation, contrast dye, and chemo can damage the organs and possibly cause other cancers. Even blood work or chemo ports can cause blood clots or infection.

I'm thankful for all those who are working diligently to find cures for the disease. God bless the doctors and nurses who press on despite the discouragement they must face every time a patient dies. Please take time to thank your medical team.

For more information about lung cancer, refer to the appendices of this book.

> *Let everything that has breath praise the* Lord*. Praise the* Lord*!*
>
> —Psalm 150:6

Chapter 29

TOO MANY OPINIONS

Dr. Davis's assistant called Chris on November 4, 2014. He and three other oncologists we'd been working with in the thoracic department had discussed Chris's situation. When they saw he had only received one round of the standard chemo, Alimta, they suggested he consider going back on it. Dr. Davis also recommended going back on crizotinib until Chris found a clinical trial.

Two days later, we saw an oncologist for the first time in the Clinical Center for Targeted Therapy at MD Anderson to discuss RXDX-101. Dr. Wentz* said Chris could start the phase I trial on December 23 in the third dose-escalation group. Only eleven patients had been tested so far in the United States, and no results had been posted. I was afraid this low dosage wouldn't work. If Chris failed the treatment, the disease would progress. The trial would require another biopsy, MRI, and CT scans. He'd have to go to Houston weekly for the first six weeks, with two days of pretesting. The first day of taking the drug, he'd have hourly blood draws and EKGs similar to the last study.

As soon as we left the doctor's office, a torrent of tears drenched my shirt. The stress of our having to make yet another decision that impacted my husband's life got to me, and I felt our life was spinning out of control.

When we got back to the hotel, I tried to regain control the best way I knew—I started contacting other oncologists for their advice.

Dr. Schaefer in Arkansas recommended we try a PD-1 or PD-L1 inhibitor, a completely different approach from another ALK inhibitor. But he didn't have any trials open for them.

Dr. Gerber from UT Southwestern recommended AT13387, which targets a heat shock protein.

Next, I contacted Dr. Jack West of cancergrace.org. He wrote,

> *I'm skeptical of giving multiple ALK inhibitors with remarkably overlapping mechanism of action, compared with chemotherapy. It may be possible to return to an agent on which the cancer previously progressed [crizotinib]. Every once in a while, the treatment is beneficial, though usually only very minimally and transiently. I suggest Alimta because there's no evidence trying a third or fourth ALK inhibitor would have any benefit. I'm more hopeful of trying a new angle rather than using a slight variant of the same treatment over and over that the cancer has already mastered.*

Convinced there had to be a simple solution everyone could agree on, I considered contacting the University of Colorado oncologist again for his opinion.

"You're searching for an answer that doesn't exist," Chris said. "No one knows what will work, as this is uncharted territory."

He was right. Instead, I referred to my previous notes from the doctor and saw he had suggested retrying Alimta.

"I don't want to take Alimta again," Chris said. "I feel that would signify the beginning of the end because I'm out of options."

I thought it would buy him time until more options developed.

All combined, nine different oncologists gave six different recommendations. How were we supposed to figure out the best plan when the doctors couldn't even agree on a plan, and Chris didn't want the treatment that several of them did agree on?

DICHOTOMY OF EMOTIONS

We finally headed home from Houston. I was driving, so after we were out of the crazy traffic and construction detours, I brought up the treatments using baseball analogies.

"Crizotinib was strike one against the cancer with a fastball. LDK378 was strike two with another fastball. X-396 was a ball that hit the batter and let the disease take a base. The cancer expects another fastball and is prepared for it. The doctors are saying we need to do a changeup and throw a curve ball. Since RXDX-101 is another inhibitor drug, I don't feel it's the right choice. We need to try something different."

Chris wasn't happy with me. He didn't want to get a port for Alimta or AT13387, even though patients I talked with who had them were glad they had one. He didn't want the reminder every time he looked in a mirror. He said, "You've been obsessed with researching treatments and asking people on the internet their opinions."

He might as well have stabbed me in the heart. *I'm spending hour upon hour trying to find statistics on various clinical trials. I'm talking with patients who have had treatments he is considering. I'm consulting with the most reliable oncologists I know to see what they recommend to help him make the best decision to save his life—and he's frustrated with me? That's the thanks I get for putting my life on hold to extend his?* Tears scalded my cheeks as my heart shattered.

He then said, "It just confuses me more, and I feel you're trying to find someone to support what you want me to do. I feel like you don't want me to do RXDX-101."

I argued, "Seeing how stressed we are going to Houston just two weeks in a row, I'm not sure we could handle weekly trips to MD Anderson for six weeks in a row for the phase I trial."

We were mentally exhausted and frustrated with Houston traffic and road closures. Our normal four-hour trip once took seven hours due to bad weather and an accident that shut down the highway. He was tired of the Houston restaurants in the medical area, numerous medical tests, appointments, long days at the cancer center, and being away from home and our local support system. The weekly blood draws would add to his stress.

I didn't tell him that if we would be in Houston during Christmas and New Year's, I couldn't stand the thought of missing time with Chad while he was home from Europe. I missed our boys so much, and not being able to spend Christmas with family was more than I could bear. To top it off, we'd also be on the road with holiday traffic.

We weren't used to being angry with each other, and I didn't know how to handle my indignation. Crying profusely, I turned up the music so he could listen while I silently fanned the flames of my smoldering resentment.

Chris curled up with a pillow against the window, trying to sleep and ignore the situation. But he didn't succeed. I glanced over later, and tears were streaming down his face.

Self-absorbed with my thoughts and emotions, I hadn't been paying attention to the music. When I saw him crying, I opened my ears and heard Al Denson singing "In the Arms of My Lord." Chris could relate to the lyrics, and they hit him hard.

Tears of compassion burst from my eyes. If there had been a place to pull off the road to hug him, I would have. Instead,

I reached over and gently placed my hand on his arm and squeezed it to let him know I loved him and was still there for him. Such was the dichotomy of emotions when dealing with cancer.

"I feel the fight go out of me a little bit more each day." He choked on his words as tears soaked his pillow.

My eyes flooded again. I cried for almost two hours while driving, angels leading the way since I could barely see the road.

"I apologize for being such a jerk," Chris said when we got home.

Hugging him tightly, I accepted his apology. "I know you're just super stressed out."

It was impossible to stay mad at my man. He wasn't perfect, but he was still the perfect husband for me.

That weekend, I put together a spreadsheet showing which doctors recommended what treatment and why, as well as the pros and cons of each, and gave it to Chris to look at. We had to process a lot of information that week, and it was overwhelming. We asked people to pray for clarity for us as we tried to make a decision.

> *"Call to Me and I will answer you, and I will tell you great and mighty things, which you do not know."*
>
> —Jeremiah 33:3

GAME PLAN DECIDED

We saw Dr. Gerber, our Dallas oncologist, on November 10. In the waiting room, I showed Chris some literature from the internet about various treatments currently available for the ALK mutation. It included the side effects of each as well as the pros and cons. He was adamant he didn't want the AT13387 that Dr. Gerber had previously mentioned.

"I'd have to get a port, and I do *not* want a port," he said.

"But all the cancer patients I've heard from that have a port are glad they got one. It makes getting chemo so much easier," I said, trying to change his mind.

"I do not want a port. Period." He was still trying to decide if he wanted to start Alimta again when they called him into the exam room.

After examining him, Dr. Gerber discussed treatment options. "If it were my family member in your position, I would recommend AT13387 plus crizotinib. I don't think an ALK inhibitor is the best option for you right now. We could keep Alimta as a backup plan. I strongly recommend getting a port, because AT13387 causes a burning sensation when it's put in a vein in the arm. The port is about the size of a dime. In one of my patients, you can't even see it. We've been seeing a 70 percent positive response with this treatment. However, to my knowledge, it hasn't been tried on anyone like you, who has failed three ALK inhibitors."

He then explained how the phase II study drug worked to attack the cancer cells. "Reports are showing that returning to a previous drug after a long period of time has still been somewhat effective. By throwing the new drug at the disease along with crizotinib, it should have a synergistic effect."

Dr. Gerber was the only doctor to sit with us and clearly define a treatment path for Chris, how the drug works, possible side effects and complications, and how he would treat them if they occurred. Although Chris wasn't comfortable with this option when Dr. Gerber had presented it to him a couple of months earlier, after processing what he said, Chris concluded this was now the best option for him.

"I think that sounds like a good plan."

What? Just fifteen minutes before in the waiting room, Chris wasn't interested in that drug and was refusing a port, and suddenly he's willing to get both? Apparently, Dr. Gerber has more clout than I do. I was a bit miffed with Chris that within just a few minutes, Dr. Gerber had completely changed my husband's mind. Apparently, my research held no validity since I didn't have a medical degree. But I agreed Dr. Gerber's suggestion was the best plan.

> *I waited patiently for the* Lord*; and He inclined to me and heard my cry. He brought me up out of the pit of destruction, out of the miry clay, and He set my feet upon a rock making my footsteps firm. He put a new song in my mouth, a song of praise to our God.*
>
> —Psalm 40:1–3

Chapter 30

FOURTH CLINICAL TRIAL

Chris spent his birthday getting a baseline echocardiogram, labs, and an eye exam per the study requirements. We also met with Rachael, the clinical trial nurse, and Chris signed the official consent form for AT13387 plus crizotinib. She assured us he wouldn't be randomized.

On November 19, he had a port inserted in the right side of his chest.

Rachael called after we got home. She apologized, then told Chris he had been randomized in the trial and wouldn't get crizotinib after all. He would just be getting AT13387 in this arm of the study. She gave him the opportunity to withdraw from the trial.

"This is the only door that's open to me," he said. "I've already done everything to get in the study, so let's just continue to move forward."

I wondered if AT13387 would work without crizotinib. I was glad, though, that he would only have to deal with side effects of one drug instead of two.

At the clinic the next day for Chris's preinfusion visit, Rachael was the first one in the door to talk to us. We could tell her mistake was bothering her immensely, and she apologized again.

"Do me a favor," Chris told her. "Forget what you told me before. We're starting over today to beat this cancer."

Appreciative for his forgiveness, she gave us her pager and private cell numbers to call her anytime. "Of the fifty-one patients enrolled to date, only eight have been on the trial drug alone [monotherapy] but have had good control of the disease," she reassured us.

After that, we were off to the infusion ward for his first chemo dose. He would get an IV infusion every week for three weeks and then have a week off.

As I drove us home, Edgar DeBoue, one of Chris's best friends, called to check on him. Chris was cheerful and laughing. Ten minutes later, he became fidgety and restless, suddenly not feeling well. Moisture glistened in the corners of his eyes.

"Cancer sucks."

This was the typical moment-by-moment emotional roller coaster for a cancer patient.

After a rough week adjusting to side effects of nausea and diarrhea, Chris finally felt like his health was stable.

At our next appointment, Dr. Gerber told us that AT13387 had shown to be effective in 60–70 percent of patients as a monotherapy. "But stats aren't important. It will either work or it won't."

CHRIS'S NEW NORMAL

The cancer roller coaster ride is humbling and not for the faint of heart or for those who are vain about their looks. Chris's body took a beating. At times he didn't look sick, so people couldn't fathom what he was going through. He worked full time until two weeks before he died. After he passed away, his supervisor told me, "I would see him every day and honestly never knew how bad he was feeling. He always had a positive, can-do attitude and a smile. I never once heard him complain."

His "new normal" was continually changing and consisted of any combination of numerous side effects, emotional ups and downs, and painful procedures. The benefits at that time—extending his life—exceeded the misery of side effects. The one common side effect he escaped was "chemo brain," also known as "chemo fog."

Oddly enough, I'm the one who experienced memory problems and cognitive dysfunction. I frequently found myself staring at my to-do list or piles of paperwork and couldn't decide where to even start. I was normally focused and task oriented, but multitasking became nearly impossible. My mind was fuzzy. I could easily remember things related to Chris and his health, but sometimes conversations and facts that weren't critical were tough to recall.

SUPER BUG

Just as Chris was starting to feel better, he had another setback on December 11. He ran a fever with a presumed urinary tract infection.

The last time we were in Houston, we had eaten lunch in MD Anderson's cafeteria. Signs stood on each table encouraging patients to seek medical attention if they run a fever over 100.5 degrees, especially if they have a port or a weak immune system. A simple infection can turn into sepsis, a life-threatening bloodstream infection. I made sure Chris read the sign.

This time he didn't argue with me about going to the hospital. We went to our local hospital since this illness wasn't cancer related.

They discovered he had *Klebsiella pneumoniae,* a super bug that had spread to his bloodstream and is commonly acquired in hospital-like settings. Patients who have IV catheters and compromised health issues are at the greatest risk from this infection, which might not respond to antibiotics. It can be fatal if not caught early. Fortunately, I didn't find out how serious it was until he was already showing improvement.

> *God is our refuge and strength, a very present help in trouble.*
>
> —Psalm 46:1

Chapter 31

OXYGEN ON ROOM AIR

Chris regained 5 pounds by the end of December, and I thought life was looking up again. I should have learned by then to not think so fast.

On January 7, 2015, Chris tested positive for the flu and was admitted to the hospital. The flu in lung cancer patients can quickly turn into deadly pneumonia. Even with a collapsed lung and illness, his oxygen level on room air remained 95–100 percent, so he didn't need supplemental oxygen.

"I feel like God has abandoned me. I've felt good only two days in the last month. How much longer will this continue?" Chris was holding back pent-up tears.

On days like that, I just held him and let him vent. He knew deep down God hadn't abandoned him.

Many times people encouraged him to stay positive. That was hard to do when he was feeling miserable, especially over a long period. He felt they didn't realize the severity of what he was dealing with every day. It was difficult to be brave and upbeat all the time. Pressured to put on a courageous face to make *them* feel better about how he was doing, he walked a fine line between facing his daily reality and remaining hopeful for a bright future. He appreciated it when people allowed him to be himself and let him know they were there for him and cared about how he was *really* doing.

STABLE SCANS

His next checkup with Dr. Gerber was January 22. Scans showed the cancer was unchanged. He said, "There's so much 'gmish' in your right lung, the radiologist can't distinguish if cancer is there or not. It's really a mess in there."

The radiologist even mentioned it appeared Chris had part of his lung removed. This wasn't the first or the last radiologist to incorrectly interpret that he'd had a lobectomy.

Chris was more energetic, his breathing exercises were improving, his coughing was decreasing, and he was gaining weight. The doctor took those as signs the treatment was working. Chris could continue in the clinical trial.

I looked at my husband and was amazed at how well he was doing, especially considering what he had been through and the usual prognosis for his disease. I saw evidence every day that God was still in the miracle business. There was no other explanation.

FRUSTRATIONS WITH HOSPITAL STAFF

Our itemized hospital bill showed a $459 charge for supplemental oxygen that Chris didn't receive during his recent hospitalization. I contacted the billing clerk and told him the bill was in error. He informed me the nurses and doctors noted, "Device: room air" when they listed Chris's oxygen level in their reports.

"Your husband didn't have a nasal cannula, but they piped oxygen into the room air."

"You're kidding, right?" I asked.

He was serious.

"May I speak with your supervisor?"

He transferred my call.

"The doctor ordered air saturation in the room," the supervisor stated.

"Are you telling me they piped oxygen into the entire room?"

"Yes."

I asked her to call me back after speaking to a medical professional for clarification.

She later returned my call, saying, "The respiratory therapist confirmed there are two ways to give patients oxygen—with a mask or room air."

It was apparent the billing staff didn't have a medical background—or common sense—and had never been around someone who needed supplemental oxygen. The supervisor interpreted the respiratory therapist's explanation the way she wanted (if she even consulted the medical professional). Maybe she didn't want to admit they were wrong and hoped in my ignorance I would believe their story.

I then called the hospital directly. I was told the nurses' notes showed Chris had a nasal cannula.

I went to the hospital to get a copy of the reports. The medical records clerk wouldn't release information to me even after I gave her the medical power of attorney with a separate HIPAA release attached as part of the same document. She insisted I needed a letter from Chris's doctor saying he was incapacitated before she could release his records to me.

"The separate HIPAA release authorization drawn up by our attorney clearly states I'm authorized to obtain his medical records even if my husband is fully competent at that time," I said.

We argued for several minutes before I asked her to check with a supervisor. While waiting on the phone to speak with her supervisor, the clerk looked at the document again and said, "Oh. This is a separate HIPAA release. This will work."

I stated calmly, "That's what I have been telling you," but I was seething inside.

After giving me the medical records, she instructed me to go down the hallway to obtain a CD of the x-rays I had requested. As soon as I walked into that department, a clerk greeted me.

"You must be here to pick up a CD."

I assumed the records clerk had told her I was on my way. She handed a CD to me without even asking my name, the patient's name, or asking for my identification. I looked at the CD, and it belonged to a female patient who was definitely not my husband. Within minutes, I had gone from one extreme to the other with customer service.

Next, I went upstairs and spoke with three nurses at the station outside the room where Chris had stayed. I told them what the billing department had said about the oxygen. They all laughed and confirmed that the hospital does *not* pipe oxygen into the room air.

"That would mean anyone in the room would be breathing the oxygen. Can you imagine what it would take to get enough oxygen piped in the room for it to benefit the patient? We don't use a nasal cannula unless the patient's oxygen saturation level drops below 92 percent."

I looked through the reports. Chris did *not* have a nasal cannula, and it was *not* listed in any of the nurses' notes.

Even though the nurses agreed with me, the billing department didn't, so I requested a grievance committee get involved. The committee saw a respiratory therapist's notes where she checked a box showing Chris had a nasal cannula. I then obtained a copy of her notes. I think she accidentally checked the wrong box, which would have been an easy error to make. Because of that one check mark, they said the charge was accurate and would not be removed.

I contacted the guest relations manager to ask the grievance committee to look at the regular attending nurses' notes. "Have them look at the entire picture for that morning in question to see that his oxygen level was 95–100 percent on room air during his entire stay. There was no medical need whatsoever for supplemental oxygen."

He ended up meeting with the president and the chief financial officer (CFO) to present Chris's medical records. They agreed the charge was in error and removed it from the bill.

Afterward, I contacted the billing supervisor to make sure they weren't charging other patients for breathing room air. If they were billing us for room air, they were probably charging all patients for it.

"You will see the charge for oxygen has been reversed," I said. "I verified with hospital staff that they do *not* pipe oxygen into the room, as you had understood it to be. Please make sure that other patients aren't being charged for oxygen when you see, 'Device used: room air.' "

"I only go by what they tell us to bill for," the supervisor said.

She wasn't convinced that I knew what I was talking about. So in my thank-you letters to the president, CFO, and guest relations manager, I explained what had transpired and asked them to educate the billing department so other patients don't get billed for oxygen when they were simply breathing room air.

Most people would have probably given up. But I'm tenacious when on a mission for justice. They messed with the wrong (or right) lady.

> *He loves righteousness and justice; the earth is full of the lovingkindness of the* Lord.
>
> —Psalm 33:5

Chapter 32

COUNTING OUR BLESSINGS

Hospital billing errors weren't the only errors I confronted. During online research, I noticed the descriptions for the ALK inhibitor drugs were suddenly showing the trials were only for squamous cell cancer. Chris had adenocarcinoma (non-small cell lung cancer).

This confused me, so I asked Dr. Gerber about it. "Is adenocarcinoma considered to be squamous cell?

"No, it's in the group for *non*-squamous cell."

"I noticed alectinib and other ALK trials are now for squamous cell on the clinicaltrials.gov website," I said. "Are they simply expanding, or is it only for squamous cell now? Or could they be typographical errors?"

"ALK inhibitors are only for non-squamous cell." He was shocked they would have it listed wrong. That could negatively affect enrollment in the trials.

I gave him the reference numbers for the trials in question, and after he looked at the website, he said they were, indeed, errors. He contacted the government website and got the information corrected.

Dr. Gerber had always seemed to appreciate the way I tried to remain informed and organized Chris's caregiving, and he treated me with respect as a member of the medical team.

IMERMAN ANGELS

Imerman Angels is an international program that recruits mentors to provide emotional support for cancer patients and their caregivers, matching them with someone going through the same type of cancer and treatment. I signed up to be a Mentor Angel and was matched with Kay in Colorado. We talked fairly often by email and sometimes by phone.

"How do you fight depression?" she asked.

"I look at how far Chris has come and how God has taken care of us every step of the way. We've been blessed by friends and family in every way imaginable. I'm thankful for each additional day that God has allowed me to share with Chris, especially when statistics say he shouldn't, couldn't, and wouldn't be here more than six to nine months. When I count my blessings, one by one, it's difficult to be depressed."

> *Rejoice always; pray without ceasing; in everything give thanks, for this is God's will for you in Christ Jesus.*
>
> —1 THESSALONIANS 5:16–18

NED A THIRD TIME

On March 19, 2015, we learned the cancer was either stable or Chris had no evidence of disease, depending on who we talked to. The radiology reports stated there was "no significant change from prior exam" and the area where the cancer was last time was "inflammatory/post radiation in origin with no evidence of tumor recurrent or metastatic disease."

"That means no evidence of disease," said Dr. Martin Dietrich, who was training to be an oncologist.

When Dr. Gerber came in, though, he wasn't as optimistic. "There may still be cancer that's stable, but it's difficult to tell because the lung is collapsed in that area, and all we can see is gray on the scans—not black or white."

We were grateful for either diagnosis. "Stable" is good and hard to achieve for a lung cancer patient, and it allowed Chris to continue on the same regimen.

Dr. Dietrich went back to the radiologist and asked him to look again at the scans. The radiologist complied, saying, "I see absolutely no evidence of disease anywhere."

My husband was a walking, talking, breathing miracle for the third time. We felt so blessed.

> *Now to Him who is able to do far more abundantly beyond all that we ask or think, according to the power that works within us, to Him be the glory in the church and in Christ Jesus to all generations forever and ever. Amen.*
>
> —Ephesians 3:20–21

Chapter 33

ANTICIPATORY ANXIETY

Chris was complaining of back pain. I noticed he kept walking with his right shoulder lower than his left shoulder. While putting ointment on his back to help with the pain, I noticed his spine was curved sideways, and he had a roll of fat on the right side of his back due to scrunching his body to the right. I worried that the changes in his spine would cause more fractures in his vertebrae.

Dr. Gerber had never seen a patient before whose body reacted this way to a collapsed lung and didn't know if that was the cause or not.

Talking with other lung cancer patients on inspire.com, I discovered other survivors also had this "dropped shoulder syndrome." One shoulder was more than two inches lower because their ribs became compressed over time after a lung was removed. Sure enough, Chris now measured two inches shorter.

He also developed "white-coat syndrome." His blood pressure and heart rate rose dramatically at his appointments versus his readings at home.

Although the May 7 CT scan showed his right lung was now almost totally collapsed, he was still chugging along. His oxygen level on room air was 99 percent, but he was coughing more.

Dr. Gerber was concerned the disease was back but was too microscopic to appear on the scans. "Since cancer isn't evident on the scans and we don't have a new trial ready to start yet, you can continue the current treatment for now," he said. "You're still benefitting from AT13387, but we need to keep an eye out for options for the future."

Increasingly brutal treatments caused Chris to develop anticipatory anxiety. Due to the smell and taste of the antiseptic, saline, and other drugs used, he felt nauseated when his port was accessed for the blood draws. Then, his anxiety increased when he sat down in the clinic waiting room. Next, he became nauseated before leaving for his appointments, thinking about the treatments he would have to endure. His blood pressure shot up at home before he left for his appointments. Finally, he had trouble sleeping the night before due to dreading the chemo treatment. He admitted he was having difficulty with the mental side of the battle.

On May 14 he got nauseated the minute he sat down for the blood draw, anticipating how bad he would be feeling by the end of the day. He went downhill from there, needing medication for nausea before, during, and after treatment.

He got sick on the way home. Fortunately, we were prepared. I continued driving calmly down the toll road while Chris vomited into the bags we had brought. He cleaned up with wet wipes and paper towels.

"Nausea is the worst feeling."

"My life sucks."

"What is God trying to teach me?"

These were the words I heard during this time. Knowing the type of life Chris led, I couldn't think of anything he needed to learn. I didn't have an answer other than, "Maybe He just wants you to encourage others through your experiences."

Chris hadn't posted a blog entry since November. He got the hint, and three days later he wrote "Living Psalm 13."

> *Psalm 13 was written by David. Each time I read it, I find myself thinking,* Wow, this is my life right now. *At the time David wrote this psalm, he was the anointed future king of Israel. Yet, there he was running for his life from King Saul, who sought to take his life. David, a man after God's own heart, was seeking refuge wherever he could find it. He was spending days and nights in dark and damp caves, never knowing when King Saul and his men would come. David was tired, exhausted, and he was seeking some answers. I can imagine David sitting alone at the top of a hill, feeling isolated from God, when he began to pour out his heart to God with the questions he'd been wrestling with.*
>
> *Most of David's questions can be summed up with, "How long, O Lord, will this continue?" David already knew his future. He would one day be the king of Israel, but he was so tired of running, he just had to ask. David asked God the questions that had been weighing heavy on his heart.*
>
> *The one thing that sticks out in this psalm is what's missing. Nowhere do I find that God answered any of David's questions. He didn't have to. In the final verse, David realized what God had already done for him. I can see David in a moment recalling the memory of his battle with Goliath and how with a single stone the giant was slain. He remembers how many times God has blessed him and rejoices.*
>
> *The reason I can relate to this psalm is that cancer has become my King Saul. It seeks to take my life. Even though I've now beaten cancer three times, I never know when it will show up again. At night when I can't sleep, I find myself questioning God.*

How long will this go on?

Why haven't you just healed me?

Sometimes I feel like I shouldn't question God's plan or will, but I don't think He's surprised by these questions. After all, if a man after God's own heart can ask these questions, why can't I? I don't get any answers either, because He doesn't need to answer.

Each time that cancer has shown its hideous face, God has provided a stone to slay the giant. I have to remind myself that God has continually laid the stones that have made the path I travel. I don't know how long this journey will last or where it will take me next. All I can do is pray that with each step I take, God has already placed the rock for me to step on.

Chris's next round of chemo was a week later. Before we left home, he took an Ativan pill for anxiety. Forty minutes later, I pulled into a school parking lot less than five minutes from the clinic, since he was feeling extremely anxious.

As soon as I put the car in park, he vomited into a bag.

"I don't want to do this anymore. I'm tired of feeling bad." Tears puddled in his eyes.

"We don't know what side effects other treatments may have," I said. I was afraid he would switch from the current treatment to something that might make him feel even worse.

By the time we got to the clinic, Chris had a migraine headache and was pale. His blood pressure was high when the nurse took his vitals, so she had him elevate his arm with the blood pressure cuff. She retook his blood pressure, and it was a little lower. She recorded the lower reading. Chris thought this was a dandy little trick to stay off medication for high blood pressure. Little did we know then that high blood pressure can damage the kidneys.

His head was throbbing.

"Could you turn out the lights while we wait for the doctor?" he asked me.

He was lying on the exam table with all the lights off when Dr. Gerber and Sharon, his nurse practitioner, walked in. I think they were concerned a brain tumor might be causing the sudden headache.

"I've had migraines before, and I'm sure that's all this is," Chris said.

It took some convincing before they would believe him. They were used to seeing him upright with a cheerful smile and attitude. You could see the concern in their eyes.

We discussed Chris's anxiety and his wanting to stop the treatment.

"It may be time for you to take a break from treatment," Dr. Gerber said. "Even though chemo drugs kill the cancer, there comes a point where the body just can't take it anymore, and the patients have to take a break to let their bodies recover."

After being in treatment for almost five years, Chris was seriously considering taking a break. In the meantime, Dr. Gerber reduced the dosage of the chemo to reduce the side effects of vomiting and anxiety.

Chris could stop treatment for up to four weeks and still stay in the trial. Just knowing he had that option relieved a lot of his anxiety. He wanted to take a vacation, and this would allow us to plan one.

The next morning, he felt so much better than usual after treatment that he was laughing. It warmed my heart to see a peek of the old Chris again.

Humble yourselves under the mighty hand of God, that He may exalt you at the proper time, casting all your anxiety on Him, because He cares for you.

—1 PETER 5:6–7

Chapter 34

A NEAR FIASCO

Chris decided to forgo the first treatment of his next cycle so we could go on vacation free from side effects. He wanted to go to Yellowstone National Park and see the Old Faithful geyser. In preparation for our vacation, I called the medical clinics in Yellowstone to find out their hours and whether or not they had supplemental oxygen if the elevation proved too much for Chris. I would rather be safe than sorry. I also mapped out the nearest hospitals around Yellowstone and Jackson Hole, Wyoming. Chris wasn't too happy with me. He wanted this vacation to be worry-free and a chance to get away from thinking about his medical issues. That wasn't an easy feat to attempt.

Three weeks earlier, I had seen a news story about a patient who wasn't allowed to fly on a commercial airline because she looked too sick. At our next appointment, I asked Dr. Gerber, "Will Chris need a letter from you clearing him to fly?"

"No, he's doing fine."

"Do they carry oxygen on board for emergencies?"

"Yes, but Mr. Haga wouldn't need it anyway."

On Saturday, July 4, just days before we were to fly to Wyoming, I read in a cancer magazine that flying in an airplane at higher altitudes can make breathing difficult for some people with lung issues. I suddenly felt the need to call American Airlines.

"My husband has lung cancer but doesn't use supplemental oxygen. If the altitude makes it hard for him to breathe, do you carry oxygen on board in case of a medical emergency?"

"What is his name and flight number? I will have someone call you back."

I gave them my phone number because I didn't want Chris to know I had called them.

The airline didn't return my call until 3:00 p.m. on Monday. Unfortunately, they called Chris instead of me and left a message.

He listened to the voice message, then asked, "Why would American Airlines be calling me?"

When I admitted what I'd done, he rolled his eyes, exasperated. The airline did *not* carry oxygen on board, and because I raised the concern, they wouldn't let Chris fly without a letter from his doctor saying he's stable for air travel without supplemental oxygen.

Panic set in. *Dr. Gerber sees patients on Mondays, but will I be able to reach him today? We leave for the airport first thing in the morning. Chris will kill me if I've ruined our vacation plans.*

I called Rachael, but she wasn't in her office. She had given us her personal cell phone number to make up for misinforming us about the clinical trial. I'd never used it, but this was a medical emergency that warranted the call—*my* life was at stake. Shaking, I explained my predicament. A godsend, she typed up a one-sentence letter on UT Southwestern letterhead and barely caught the doctor for his signature before he left to catch an airplane. If the airline had called just fifteen minutes later, we would have had a fiasco. Within thirty minutes, Rachael faxed the letter to me. I then faxed it to American Airlines, and they approved it.

We arrived at the airport on July 7, 2015, able to celebrate our thirty-first wedding anniversary still in wedded bliss.

We enjoyed our vacation in Yellowstone. Chris did extremely well with the altitude, although he got winded one time when walking up an incline to our car at around 8,000 feet elevation. It took him a couple of minutes to recover.

"We are *not* checking my oxygen level or pulse." (Yes, I had an oximeter in my purse.) In defiance of his condition, he started the engine and drove to our next destination.

Chris was in his element—taking photographs of nature. We watched bison walk in front of our bumper. He spotted a momma black bear and her cub a short distance from the side of the road. Ignoring my mother's instructions before we left Texas, my *National Geographic* photographer wannabe rolled down his window to get some great shots of the bear looking for ants on a downed tree. Four pounces and she could have had a really filling breakfast.

My favorite place was Schwabacher's Landing, a popular photography spot on the Snake River. Chris took me there three times to catch the Grand Teton mountain range in morning, afternoon, and dusk lighting. Tourists miss this spot if they don't know where to look for it. As I explored farther down the path alone, Chris stayed near the trailhead taking photos. The altitude and constant activity had worn him down, and he was losing stamina.

I watched him gazing at the Grand Tetons, soaking in the view as long as he could. He had seen all he needed through the camera lens. Now he was savoring the splendor with his own eyes.

This may be the last time he will ever see such majestic grandeur this side of heaven.

I didn't want to leave and face our reality again.

I will lift up my eyes to the mountains; from where shall my help come? My help comes from the Lord, who made heaven and earth.

—Psalm 121:1–2

Chapter 35

THE LAST BULLET

Chris had scans performed before our vacation. We put off reading the results until getting back from the Grand Tetons. That was a wise choice. I was proud of myself for not sneaking a peek; it would have ruined our escape.

When we read the CT scan report, it frightened the bejeebers out of us. Everything spelled bad news: no aerated right lung, left ventricular hypertrophy (LVH), tortuous thoracic aorta, abrupt cut off to the right main artery, ground-glass nodules in the left lung (his *good* lung), small pericardial effusion, and central bronchi with rapid cut off.

We were scheduled to see the nurse practitioner, but I requested to see Dr. Gerber instead to ask questions about the scans and plan our options, since we assumed the cancer had returned and Chris would be kicked out of the trial.

At our appointment on July 16, Dr. Gerber greeted us with, "I know you've read the CT report and it sounds very scary, but let me tell you what I'm seeing." He was upset the radiologist posted such a terrifying report online before our appointment and requested we send a letter with our initial reactions so he could get the policy changed.

He then opened up the previous CT scan plus the one just completed and put them side by side on his computer monitor. "Most of what was written was because two different radiologists reviewed the last two scans, and everything noted by the last radiologist was there in the previous scan. They just had different ways of looking at things."

He patiently explained each condition to us as I rapidly jotted down everything he said.

"LVH is a thickening of the muscle around the heart because it's working harder. We don't need to treat this, and it won't keep him out of clinical trials. The thoracic aorta is curved due to changes in the organ structure caused by the compressed lung. The abrupt cut off to the right main artery has been there before. The nodules are too small to biopsy to see if they're cancerous. The radiologist shows one grew by only 0.33 millimeters. They shouldn't be able to report decimal points for millimeters. The pericardial effusion is fluid around the heart. The central bronchi is cut off due to seven nodes in the mediastinum, ranging from three millimeters to nine millimeters. It's also caused by the collapsed lung."

He continued, "There's not unequivocal evidence of progression of disease. The new nodules are so small they can't be biopsied and would have to be surgically removed to determine if they are malignant—which we won't do." He didn't want to risk having Chris's only working lung collapse during an invasive procedure. "The changes aren't significant enough to stop the trial. I don't go just by the scans. I look to see how the patient is doing overall when I make decisions. You're doing well on the trial and are much improved from when you started it. There's no assurance you would do this well on another drug."

Last, the doctor talked about a couple of other options to consider. "Nivolumab, an immunotherapy, is currently FDA approved for squamous cell lung cancer, but it has only a 30 percent response rate. I'll see if your insurance will pay for it.

Sometimes they will, even if you don't have the specific cancer type it's approved for. Although I don't know when, we're also supposed to get alectinib that would be open to anyone with ALK, regardless of what previous treatments had been given."

"Alimta is still an option we're keeping in our back pocket," I reminded him.

SLIDESHOW

Chris and I had discussed funeral plans in the past, and he approved the eulogy that I had written for him. He had given me his favorite scenery photos and asked me to create a slideshow presentation for his funeral. After our recent vacation, I asked him for his favorite photos from Wyoming to add.

Earlier in the year, I had heard the song "If You Could See Me Now" by Kim Noblitt and imagined it being sung at Chris's funeral. The lyrics were about being healed and sitting at Jesus' feet in heaven. I had purchased the CD and added the song to the PowerPoint presentation. I played the slideshow with Chris sitting next to me in front of my computer. As he saw and heard it for the first time, tears spilled down his face. The combination of wonderful shared memories with the powerful lyrics set to gorgeous music overwhelmed me too. The slideshow finished with one of my favorite photos of Chris holding his camera in Yellowstone National Park. He burst into tears. It hit me just then that the next time I would see the slideshow would probably be at his funeral. I leaned over and held him in my arms as we bawled, united by our love and sorrow.

HEART-WRENCHING TALK

It was mid-August. Chris had been coughing hard for more than a week. When he came home from work, I could tell he didn't feel well.

"Something's going on. I don't feel right," he said.

He pulled only 2,000 on the incentive spirometer that evening. With his breathing capacity worse, he was considering changing cancer treatment. He was short of breath, had lost weight, and was hoarse—symptoms of lung cancer. Unfortunately, his scans were now every twelve weeks instead of every eight. We would have to wait four more weeks to get a look at what was going on.

Two weeks later, he coughed so forcefully he vomited into the kitchen sink. He felt awful and was depressed. "I feel like I'm backsliding," he said.

That night he couldn't sleep. I got up during the night and found him sitting in the living room recliner. He was silently sobbing. "How much more does God want me to endure? I feel like I'm dying. I never wanted you to have to watch me suffer. I think this is the beginning of the end. It will be all downhill from here."

It was heart-wrenching to hear him talk like that. I cried as I held him in my arms, fearing his prediction was right. *Please, Lord, don't let this be the end. I'm not ready to let him go.*

I sent Chris back to bed and closed the door while I went upstairs to sleep. I wanted to be far enough away that his coughing wouldn't keep me awake but close enough to hear if he needed me. He coughed hard for another two hours before he fell asleep.

I stayed awake for hours, tossing and turning. I tried to turn my worries into prayer but was unsuccessful. I was so tired. I tried David's war cry in 1 Samuel 17:47, "The battle is the LORD's," to remind myself who was in control. My fears calmed down, and I found peace, thinking about the good things and miracles God had done in our lives.

Reminded that our problems are opportunities for God to show His power, I fell asleep, praying for another miracle.

I cried out to God for help; I cried out to God to hear me. When I was in distress, I sought the Lord; at night I stretched out untiring hands and my soul refused to be comforted. I remembered you, O God, and I groaned; I mused, and my spirit grew faint. You kept my eyes from closing; I was too troubled to speak. . . . Then I thought, "To this I will appeal: the years of the right hand of the Most High." I will remember the deeds of the Lord*; yes, I will remember your miracles of long ago. I will meditate on all your works and consider all your mighty deeds. Your ways, O God, are holy. What god is so great as our God? You are the God who performs miracles; you display your power among the peoples.*

—Psalm 77:1–4, 10–14 NIV

CHANGE IN TREATMENT PLAN

Chris was exhausted by midmorning on September 3. "I feel worse today than I've felt in a long time. We have to do something different quickly," he said. He was scheduled to start his eleventh cycle of chemo that day.

Based on how Chris felt, Dr. Gerber agreed the treatment had run its course. "It's time to change strategy."

Alectinib still was not FDA approved, and there weren't any trials for it within easy driving distance. We needed the wheels of government to turn a little faster. Alimta was the only feasible option available. It was time to get the last bullet out of Chris's back pocket, put it in the chamber, pull the trigger, and pray it hit the mark. We prayed the standard chemo would give Chris time for the FDA to approve alectinib so it could be dispensed locally without a clinical trial.

This would be the first time in over four years that Chris wasn't in a clinical study. As part of exiting the trial, he'd have an echocardiogram, CT scan, and brain MRI. Those would show what we were dealing with and get a baseline before starting Alimta.

Alimta was the same chemo Chris had in February 2011. It helped stop the cancer, but he ended up in the hospital with an almost nonexistent immune system. It's frequently used as a maintenance chemo and has fewer side effects than the harsher chemotherapies. Chris had to delay starting it for a week while he took medications in preparation. This also gave his body time to rest before starting a chemo known to affect his blood counts.

IN DESPAIR

When doing his breathing exercises that same evening, Chris was now reaching only 1,750. I found him at 2:00 a.m. sitting in the recliner again, crying in despair. "I'm beginning to wonder if I will even make it to Thursday to start my new treatment."

I wrapped my arms around Chris and wept with him. These middle-of-the-night meetings were making us feel hopeless. I was terrified at how fast he appeared to be going downhill in both his body and spirit. *Is he just going to give up?* I felt helpless trying to console him. I needed someone to console *me*.

After my emotions settled down, I asked him a daunting question, as I wanted to make sure I followed his wishes. "If anything happens and you quit breathing, do you want to be resuscitated?"

"Yes."

Thank you, Lord. He hasn't given up yet.

FUNERAL DIRECTIVES

Two days later, Chris handed me a document he had typed. It was his updated directive for his funeral. I had seen it before, but the thought that he updated it that Saturday morning meant he truly thought the end was near.

He gave a list to me of things to do after his death, which included posting his final blog entry "A Good Ride." He told me what to do with his truck, who to contact at work, and how to protect the boys' inheritance should I remarry. *That* was tough to read. The thought of being married to anyone but Chris ripped my heart out.

It was so like him to try to take as much of the burden off my shoulders as possible. He made small repairs at home and within the next two months had all the windows and exterior doors replaced so I wouldn't have to deal with it after he died. He even looked up the value of his truck so I would know how much to sell it for.

Chad had just finished a big race in Europe. Shane had graduated from Discipleship Training School in Mexico and was planning to return home. Although there's never a good time to break bad news, we deliberately delayed posting anything about Chris's condition because we knew it could upset our sons and cause them to worry. If Chad lost concentration during a race, it could end in catastrophe.

We called our boys and told them we felt the cancer had returned so they could be mentally prepared. They took the news in stride, knowing it was always a possibility the disease would return again.

Chris wrote on his CaringBridge page:

> *Once again we find ourselves with heavy hearts. We have cried the tears and made the phone calls that needed to be made. We are still praying for and expecting a miracle. Yesterday is gone, and tomorrow is yet to come. We are doing our best to focus on today.*

> *In the morning, O Lord, You will hear my voice; in the morning I will order my prayer to You and eagerly watch.*
>
> —Psalm 5:3

Chapter 36

FATIGUE AND DEPRESSION

We got the results of the scans, and it appeared we caught the progression early. The other good news was that being off the AT13387 gave Chris's creatinine level a chance to return to normal, so his kidneys were functioning well.

Chris received his first dose of Alimta on September 10, 2015. Four days later, I found him reading his Bible at 2:00 a.m. in the living room. He was disheartened again, trying to console himself by reading Psalms. "I'm afraid my body is getting too weak to beat this."

Fatigue was already plaguing Chris before starting Alimta. One of the major side effects of this drug is also fatigue, so he was frustrated with his lack of energy. He was thankful his supervisor let him work from home.

I wouldn't let Chris drive anywhere because of the extreme fatigue. I was also afraid he would have a bad coughing spell that could cause him to pass out while driving.

As we were getting ready for church on Sunday morning, he approached me, crying. "Be sure to drive extra carefully to church. Satan is trying to keep me from going," he said.

He struggled to breathe and could barely move, but he was determined to go worship the Lord. Although we made it to church, Chris was exhausted. He only stood for the Scripture reading. He didn't have the energy to stand while the congregation sang. When we returned home, he slept the rest of the afternoon.

Why did Chris feel so strongly he needed to be in church? He could have easily stayed home, read his Bible, watched services on TV, or listened to sermons on the radio. There's something powerful about gathering in His name with other believers in worship. The Holy Spirit is multiplied in the midst of us. Most basic of all, Chris wanted to honor God.

> *"For where two or three have gathered together in My name, I am there in their midst."*
>
> —Matthew 18:20

One morning I called Dr. Gerber's nurse to ask a question about Chris's steroid schedule. Melissa returned my call while I was at the grocery store.

"How is he doing?" she asked.

That's all it took to have me standing in a puddle of tears in the middle of the store. After hearing what was going on with him, she suggested he see their palliative care physician to get help with managing the side effects of weight loss, anxiety, sleeplessness, and depression.

Surprisingly, Chris was willing. The previous month had been rough for him. Coughing spells were so forceful they caused him to lose whatever he had recently eaten. Loss of appetite caused him to lose 9 pounds in two weeks. His respirations were shallower and faster. His oxygen level went down to 92 percent during a walking test. Breathing exercises reflected he was losing lung capacity. He was beaten down mentally and physically. It was difficult to see him struggling.

The palliative care doctor quickly assessed Chris's physical as well as mental state. "Describe a good day," she said.

"It's been so long ago, I can't remember."

"That's very telling."

My heart broke to know he didn't have *any* good days. I turned away to inconspicuously dry my eyes before the teardrops leaked down my cheeks.

This wonderful doctor prescribed mirtazapine to help improve his appetite, mood, nausea, depression, and insomnia.

On CaringBridge, I wrote:

Please pray specifically for improvements in fatigue, restful sleep, appetite, nausea, blood counts, heart rate, blood pressure, and for this new treatment to work. Also please pray for the mental aspect of this journey, as it's a mental battle as well as a physical one.

Be merciful to me, LORD, for I am faint; O LORD, heal me, for my bones are in agony. My soul is in anguish. How long, O LORD, how long?

—PSALM 6:2–3 NIV

Chapter 37

PRAYERS ANSWERED

Having witnessed God's healing numerous times already, we knew He could heal Chris. But we were losing confidence this was His plan. Trusting in God isn't an insurance policy to prevent bad things from happening; otherwise, everyone would selfishly sign up for religion. We stayed devoted to Him, knowing He might not answer our prayers the way we wanted.

During this time, we were depending on others to pray for us to trust God would restore Chris's health once more. It was hard to look beyond what we were experiencing to seeing what God saw for the future.

My brother Barrick sent us a note and scripture as encouragement:

> *On those days when your faith seems lost, all used up, or hopeless, remember there are those of us out here whose faith has not been stirred or shaken. We continue to remember God has continually worked miracles for both of you that can't be explained otherwise. It's important when we pray that we pray with faith it will be done. If we pray with the feeling that it's hopeless, we're not praying with faith.*

Faith is not just knowing that God can *do it, it's knowing He* will *do it.*

When He entered the house, the blind men came up to Him, and Jesus said to them, "Do you believe that I am able to do this?" They said to Him, "Yes, Lord." Then He touched their eyes, saying, "It shall be done to you according to your faith." And their eyes were opened.

—MATTHEW 9:28–30

God continued to put the right person and treatment in the right place at the right time. Chris's health improved just one week after starting mirtazapine. He slept much better and had more energy throughout the day. He gained almost one pound each day. His cough practically disappeared. He started driving. His breathing exercises, heart rate, blood pressure, oxygen level, and respirations improved.

I stood in the kitchen one afternoon as he napped in his recliner. I watched him breathe and compared his respirations to mine. His chest was rising and falling with mine without struggle. I never thought simply watching my husband breathe would give me such peace of mind. We take so much for granted.

He was able to walk around the block—sometimes even twice. He went out with friends and was eating well. He fixed an exterior flood light fixture. He was laughing and joking again. And he was smiling. My Chris was back.

Weeping may endure for a night but joy comes in the morning.

—PSALM 30:5 NIV

The CT scan on October 19 showed Alimta was working. The nodules had decreased in size, which explained why Chris was feeling better. He was doing so well, he even quit taking the prescription cough medicine he had been on for a year. We believed God was going to give us a miracle again.

The following week, Chris wrote "Have I Been a Fool?"

Most Christians don't like having their faith challenged. I'll admit to being one of them. I've always been more of a "let my walking do my talking" kind of guy. As I've said many times before, God and I have had many one-sided discussions about the purpose of the journey I'm on. The only time God has chosen to give me any type of an answer, it was, They are watching. *He has yet to disclose to me who "they" are. I believe "they" are just people who know I'm a Christian and are watching to see how I respond to my journey and whether my faith still holds.*

The reason this has come up in my mind is that I'm now fighting active lung cancer for the fourth time. We've been praying for complete healing for five years now. Instead of healing, we receive another diagnosis of recurring disease. I can't help but believe some of the people who are watching have to think I'm foolish to continue to believe there's a god who can or will heal me. After all, the Psalms are full of passages where David's faith is ridiculed. Even Jesus was mocked while on the cross. Why should I be surprised if there are people questioning my faith in God?

To keep it real, I'll confess to having asked myself multiple times this past month if I was being foolish to believe God would heal me. There have been several nights I've stayed awake asking God where He is and imploring Him to show up. Yes, I freely admit to having fallen. One thing I've noticed in those times is that God isn't the one who has moved. It's always me who isn't where he's supposed to be. It's the times I've fallen that I find it easiest to worship God. I'm already down on my face before Him. Don't judge the absence of God by the times I've fallen, but judge the presence of God by the times that, thanks to His unfathomable grace, I've been able to stand.

Have I been a fool? I don't think so. In the Bible, we're instructed to work out our faith. In these last five years, I've come to believe that God allows trials to assist us in working out that faith. God doesn't mind the hard questions we ask. He expects them. While reading Psalm 37, I was reminded that my steps have been established by the Lord. Even when I fall, I won't be hurled headlong, because He's the One who is holding my hand.

I'm thankful that through this journey, what I believe has been transformed into faith.

"For I am the LORD *your God, who upholds your right hand, who says to you, 'Do not fear, I will help you.' "*

—ISAIAH 41:13

Chapter 38

DURABLE MEDICAL EQUIPMENT RUNAROUND

We had a pleasant experience with XYZ Healthcare* the previous November when they delivered a nebulizer for Chris's breathing treatments. It was now past time to replace its filter. I placed an order using the part number from the original paperwork. A week later, a customer service representative with this national supplier of durable medical equipment (DME) informed me I had a five-cent co-pay, 10 percent of a forty-eight-cent filter.

"We've met our out-of-pocket expenses for the year, so we have a zero co-pay," I said.

Since it was such a small amount, the rep said she'd go ahead and ship the order. A few hours later, I received a call from a different rep. She was adamant the patient needed a face-to-face meeting with the doctor before they could fill the order for the filter. After I said Chris had an appointment scheduled the next day with his doctor and could get the prescription, she suddenly changed her story and said it didn't need the doctor's approval after all. Then she said, "There's no out-of-pocket expense, but we need a credit card number to protect our asset." When I wouldn't give her my credit card number, she claimed she couldn't process the order without a credit card number on file. At my request, she transferred me to her supervisor, who tried to intimidate me to give my credit card number. Again, I refused. I didn't trust them.

After those conversations, I found hundreds of online reviews for this company—all deplorable. The Better Business Bureau gave them an "F" rating. The company failed to deliver supplies critical for sustaining life and made unauthorized charges to credit cards on file. Patients had difficulty getting their money back, even when they didn't owe it.

I called our insurance company and verified they would pay 100 percent of the cost. They had no record of XYZ contacting them to verify our co-pay.

The following morning I spoke with two more reps and a supervisor at XYZ, who all asserted our insurance pays only 90 percent. They finally shipped a filter, twice, but they sent the wrong part both times.

When I called to see if the correct filter had shipped, my order had been deleted. The clerk who reentered the order informed me they don't require a credit card number to ship. "We bill the insurance company."

The correct filter arrived twenty-three days after I placed the original order. Thank goodness this wasn't a life-or-death situation.

A few days later, I received a check from our insurance company for forty-eight cents because XYZ wouldn't accept assignment. So now I had to turn around and pay the forty-eight cents to the DME company. They were apparently determined to get my credit card number. Stubborn as a mule, I sent a check.

After that experience, I researched other DME companies in our network and read customer reviews. I found another company just ten minutes from our home that had good reviews and put their information in my binder for future reference. I learned to not leave it up to a doctor's office to choose the DME company for us again.

> *A false balance is an abomination to the* Lord, *but a just weight is His delight.*
>
> —Proverbs 11:1

Chapter 39

CAREGIVERS FOR THE CAREGIVER

I'd been having trouble with my right shoulder for almost a year and needed surgery. *But when? Who would take care of Chris? Who would take care of me?* I saw my window of opportunity when Chris's health improved again, and both our sons were going to be home. Shane had returned from mission work in Mexico, and Chad was in his off season.

Dr. Douthit performed surgery on October 21 to repair my rotator cuff, a torn bicep, frozen shoulder, and a frayed labrum. I was in for a long initial recovery plus physical therapy. The roles were suddenly reversed. Chris immediately became my caregiver, and I was the patient.

Forbidden to move my arm and shoulder, I required assistance showering and dressing. Chris went with me to get my hair cut and learned how to curl my hair. Try as he might, this manly man was all thumbs when it came to using hot rollers and a curling iron. He was so frustrated, as were our boys when I recruited their help, that I finally had to ask my female friends to curl my hair.

Chris was wonderful about filling the ice machine for my shoulder therapy and making sure I took my medications on schedule. Chad and Shane took care of the cooking and the dishes while they were home so Chris could have enough energy to take care of me and still get his regular job done. Then both boys left for around a month. Shane went to Mexico to do more missionary work, building homes for families in need. Chad went to Colorado to meet a woman named Kate, whom he had met online through mutual friends playing matchmaker.

I didn't want to wear Chris out taking care of me, so I enlisted help with meals. People provided home-cooked meals and gift cards for restaurants. Both were appreciated. Mom dusted, vacuumed, did laundry, ironed my shirts, and washed dishes. Friends took turns taking me to physical therapy three times a week since I wasn't allowed to drive.

After just a week of taking care of me, Chris readily admitted he would prefer to be the patient than the caregiver. I, too, preferred my original role.

I have learned to be content whatever the circumstances.

—PHILIPPIANS 4:11 NIV

Chapter 40

RANDOM FEVERS AND FRUSTRATING HOSPITALIZATION

Chris should have never mentioned he preferred to be the patient. He soon got his wish. Within a three-day span, he went to the ER twice because of a high fever and low oxygen and was hospitalized the second time. A doctor suspected there might be pockets of infection in the fluid around his right lung. "We can inject something that will loosen up the pockets to allow excess fluid to be drained, which could help reinflate the lung," he suggested.

We didn't feel the lung would ever reinflate based on what his oncologists had said. The radiation fibrosis permanently damaged and collapsed part of the lung, and the tumor collapsed the rest of it—not the fluid. It had been totally collapsed now for several months, and we couldn't imagine it would be healthy enough to reinflate, short of a miracle.

While I had extra time on my hands in the hospital, I began clearing out some old emails and came across one from 2013 that included my spreadsheet correlating Chris's fevers of unknown origin with CT scans and high creatinine levels. I had forgotten about that spreadsheet. Because of my finding, his medical chart includes his allergy to CT contrast. Once they started giving Chris 1 liter of saline after the scans and chemo, he quit running the high temperatures.

Since starting on Alimta, Chris's creatinine had slowly increased over time, but he hadn't received extra fluids after scans, and he received only 500 cc (cubic centimeters) after chemo. The previous week, his creatinine was higher than it had ever been when tested during his fevers. Now that he was receiving fluids in the hospital, his creatinine was closer to normal, and his fever disappeared. I was seeing a correlation again.

Saturday evening, November 7, I told the nurse we hadn't heard the results of the CT scan. The hospitalist had gone home before the results were posted, so the nurse called the doctor and read the results to him. The doctor then called Chris and said, "No blood clot was found, and the scan looks about the same as the October 19 scans. There's no clear reason for fever and low oxygen."

Chris's breathing exercises were now back at his normal level, so I asked his nurse to see what his oxygen level was on room air. Was he going to need to go home with oxygen or not? Fifteen minutes after removing the nasal cannula, his oxygen level was 97 percent. That lifted his spirits.

Sunday morning, the hospitalist and oncologist on call said they suspected empyema, a collection of pus in the fluid around the lung that can get infected. "The pleural effusion is thickening and forming a rind," the hospitalist said. "We could open up the outer lining of the lung and clean it out. We'll have the CVTS [cardiovascular thoracic surgeon] talk to you to help make a decision about getting a sample of the fluid."

Sunday afternoon, I was tired of being cooped up in the hospital room with football on TV. I hate football. I didn't have much confidence we would see the CVTS or get dismissed before Monday. I felt we had been stranded for the weekend with no active treatment taking place. Chris hadn't felt bad at all that week, even with the fevers, and his vitals were good enough to go home.

I hadn't showered in four days. I was wearing clothes two days at a time and had no more clean clothes with me. We hadn't even washed up that day for fear we would miss the doctor. I hadn't been sleeping well since my shoulder surgery. I slept even worse at the hospital, sleeping upright in a hard chair with my arm in a sling.

We weren't getting any answers or communication, and I reached my breaking point. After crying from exhaustion and frustration for an hour, I asked a woman at the front desk when the doctor would be in. I calmed down when she said he would be by in about an hour.

The CVTS disagreed with the on-call oncologist. The CVTS felt that chemo caused the fevers—not empyema. "The ribs are so close together now due to the collapsed lung, I don't think we could squeeze a catheter between the ribs," he said. "Another option would be antibiotics, although it could be hard for the antibiotics to reach the isolated spaces. The small pockets of fluid might not be as loculated as we think, but they may have turned to gel and are too thick to suck out even if we use an agent to help liquefy it."

"Would my lung reinflate?" Chris asked.

"No. It's not unreasonable to sample the fluid, but it's *not* my first recommendation. I recommend you do *not* do any procedure at this time because there's a chance it would not give us an answer, and there's risk of introducing an infection anytime a procedure is done." After looking at the CT scans back to 2012, he showed us there was very little change in the pleural effusion.

A little later, a CVTS fellow came in to practice getting medical history and giving recommendations. He didn't know what the CVTS had told us earlier. His opinion matched the CVTS's, and he thought Chris could be dismissed.

When the hospitalist came back in, she said, "The CVTS told me to schedule a meeting with Interventional Radiology, and he wants a sample."

We were adamant that wasn't what we had been told or agreed to. The hospitalist didn't want to dismiss Chris until we met with Interventional Radiology the next day for a procedure.

Chris turned beet red in the face. I could see his frustration building as he thought about how to respond. He took a deep breath before calmly, but firmly, responding, "I don't feel the risk is worth the reward. I don't see a need to spend another night in the hospital. I'll discuss our options with my personal oncologist this week. I want to go home."

"I'll document you elected to leave against my medical advice," she said.

She did, and we did.

A fool always loses his temper, but a wise man holds it back.

—PROVERBS 29:11

Chapter 41

A SMALL MIRACLE

"I'm running a fever."

You've got to be kidding. Really? I had felt Chris's forehead before going to bed, and his temperature was normal. In just thirty minutes, it shot up to 101.5 degrees. We finally got it to come down with acetaminophen and cold wash cloths. We should have gone to the ER, but we just couldn't make ourselves go again that night. He had only been home from the hospital six days.

He ran a fever again on the next day, but we got it to go back down. Chris was supposed to speak the next night at our local hospital for Lung Cancer Awareness Month, he was scheduled for chemo on Thursday, plus I had three physical therapy appointments scheduled that week. We didn't have time for him to be hospitalized again. The pulmonologist had said if he developed a fever again over the weekend, he would need a thoracentesis to draw fluid from the lung and test for infection. It was apparent what needed to be done.

How am I going to get my range of motion back if I have to keep rescheduling my physical therapy? I'm embarrassed to admit I had a moment of resentment. I don't know if it was directed toward Chris or the cancer. *My life revolves around him. Just when I think I can finally do something to take care of myself, his needs take precedence once again.*

But I quickly snapped out of my private pity party when I realized Chris would love to worry only about shoulder rehab instead of lung cancer.

He had the thoracentesis on Wednesday. He didn't have empyema, and no cancer cells or active infections were detected in the fluid.

"I don't think it would be a good idea to drain the fluid with a catheter, and it wouldn't work in your case," the pulmonologist said. He looked at all of Chris's CT scans over the last few years and compared them with the scan taken in the hospital on November 7. "In March, it was evident your right lung was totally collapsed. A small area of your right lung has actually opened back up some time between the October 19 and November 7 CT scans." He pointed the area out to us on the monitor. "I feel the chemo has reduced the cancer in the lung and allowed it to reinflate a little. I'm very surprised at the resilience of your lung. A lung that's been collapsed for as long as yours has, especially due to radiation fibrosis, doesn't normally open back up."

We counted that as a small miracle. Chris's faith had moved a mountain.

> *"I tell you the truth, if you have faith as small as a mustard seed, you can say to this mountain, 'Move from here to there' and it will move. Nothing will be impossible for you."*
>
> —Matthew 17:20 NIV

Chapter 42

LAST MAN STANDING

Chris was hospitalized again on December 6 after running a fever for four days. I looked through my notes to see if there was a pattern for when he developed the fevers in relation to chemo. Being detail oriented paid off again. My charting showed that when he was on steroids for the chemo and antibiotics for the fever, the fever went away. When he stopped those medications, the fever reappeared. When I told the oncologist the pattern I found, he thought the chemo was causing the fevers since they couldn't find a medical cause. He had one other patient that developed a high temperature when on chemo, and the fevers stopped when chemo was stopped. He dismissed Chris with a prescription to take an antibiotic for six weeks.

On October 9, 2015, nivolumab became FDA approved for non-small cell lung cancer. Now called Opdivo, it's frequently advertised on television. On December 15, 2015, the FDA approved alectinib. We now had two more spare bullets without going through a clinical trial.

We learned that our friend Bill Haines had passed away on December 29. He began treatment a month before Chris did, and they had gone through radiation together. His death hit us hard. He was the last surviving friend we knew from MD Anderson. Once a strong man and an assistant police chief, he had now succumbed to lung cancer. Chris was the last man standing. How much longer could he make it?

It's probably difficult for people who don't face a terminal diagnosis daily to understand the constant anxiety that can explode without warning when another friend with your diagnosis passes away. We were in this battle together. Every time a friend with the disease died, they took a part of us with them. Bit by bit, our hope for long-term survival was being chewed up. In our world, there was no "post-traumatic" stress—it was ongoing. We grieved the loss while wondering if death would strike our home next.

How did we handle what could have become debilitating anxiety? We focused on doing whatever it took to keep Chris alive. We put one foot in front of the other like warriors and marched on to the battlefield. And we prayed. Then we tried to make the most of each day while waiting for the answer to prayer.

> *Do not be anxious about anything, but in everything, by prayer and petition, with thanksgiving, present your requests to God. And the peace of God, which transcends all understanding, will guard your hearts and your minds in Christ Jesus. Finally, brothers, whatever is true, whatever is noble, whatever is right, whatever is pure, whatever is lovely, whatever is admirable—if anything is excellent or praiseworthy—think about such things.*
>
> —PHILIPPIANS 4:6–8 NIV

Chapter 43

LOVE AND THE MIRACLE MAN, JR.

Chad was smitten with Kate. He wanted us to meet her and asked if she could stay with us in December. I knew they must be serious about each other.

The more I got to know Kate, the more I understood why Chad had grown to love her so quickly. She was everything he had been looking for in a wife. Kate fit in well with our family, and we all quickly grew to love her. There was no doubt in our minds that she was the right woman for Chad.

On December 30, 2015, during a moonlit stroll around a popular park in McKinney, Chad asked her to marry him.

"Are you serious?" she asked.

What is it about the Haga men that their proposals aren't taken seriously?

Fortunately, she only asked the question once before accepting his proposal. They bought their engagement and wedding rings a few days later, just one day before Chad left for Spain for training camp and Kate flew back to Colorado.

THE ACCIDENT

It was Saturday, January 23, 2016. Chris walked into the living room with his cell phone.

"I just received a phone call that shows it's from the Netherlands. They didn't leave a message. It must be a scam." Just as he finished the sentence, he received another phone call from the same number.

"Chad's team is based in the Netherlands," I said. "You'd better answer it."

It was the team director.

"The team had finished their training ride, and some cyclists were hit by a car that crossed over the line coming toward them. Six riders were injured, including Chad. Since they were in the middle of nowhere, Chad was taken by helicopter to the nearest hospital with a neck wound and is in surgery right now. His injuries appear to be non-life threatening. He was helping other teammates out after the accident until someone pointed out his neck was bleeding."

We were shaken from the news, but the director sounded as if Chad's injuries weren't that serious. As the news sunk in that he was hit at least partly head-on, my knees became wobbly, just as when Chris told me there were tumors in his lung. Chris was distraught. He sat in his recliner and cried. Although he didn't say it, I think he momentarily felt guilty for encouraging Chad to pursue his dream of cycling. I got down on my knees beside him, held his hands, and prayed for Chad and his teammates.

After we pulled ourselves together, Chris called Kate to let her know. She had already heard the news and was making plans to fly to Spain to be with Chad. If she hadn't already won my heart, that would have done the trick. God had brought this wonderful woman into Chad's life at just the right moment.

In a private conversation with Kate just a month earlier, I confided to her that I worried about something happening to

Chad in Europe, and we wouldn't be able to fly there to help him due to Chris's health. The thought of our son being alone in a strange hospital in a foreign country, in pain and confused, was almost more than I could bear.

Then we had to tell Shane. He was shocked to hear his older brother had been injured in a horrific accident so far from home, but he quickly joined us in spreading the news to friends and family and keeping them updated as we learned more about Chad's condition and progress. Then Optum, Chad's previous team in the United States, generously offered to fly Shane to Spain to be with him. Shane jumped at the chance. He assisted in Chad's recovery, and despite the circumstances, it was a blessing to both of them to spend this time together as best friends one last time before Chad's marriage.

The crash was more horrendous than we had thought. The driver was a British woman driving in Spain on the wrong side of the road. She came around a blind curve from the opposite direction at the same time as the team. She hit the team head-on at a fairly high speed for both car and bicycles. Photos of the accident scene showed a mangled car, a bashed-in windshield, broken bikes, and one bike still underneath the front of the car. It's a miracle no one was killed.

Chad required almost one hundred stitches to repair veins and arteries in his neck and face. His eye socket was fractured, and he had multiple contusions and abrasions across his body. To come *face-to-face* with a car going probably 40–50 mph and not break his neck, have major internal injuries, or even get a concussion was nothing short of miraculous. I called him "My Miracle Man, Jr." We continued to count our blessings.

Knowing that many of our friends and family were praying for Chad, his teammates, and our family gave us a sense of peace. We gave God the glory for saving his life. With the news coverage and numerous interviews, Chad was able to share his faith all over the world.

He was in the intensive care unit for a few days, and he called us the day after the accident.

"How do you feel?" I asked.

"I feel like I got hit by a car," he said in a voice we barely recognized.

Throughout his ordeal, he maintained his witty sense of humor, which he got from his father. Humorous tweets from the ICU gained media attention. Chad was dismissed from the hospital five days after the accident and returned to training less than two weeks later. Two months after the accident, he was racing again.

CHAD'S ARTICLE

After his dad passed away, Chad wrote an article "Chad Haga Journal: My Mobile Think-Tank" published August 1, 2016, on VeloNews.com. Here's a clip:

> *The good news is that all the turmoil this year—the most trying of my life by leaps and bounds—has not cost me my desire to race. Instead, I've doubled down. Hagas are fighters. My dad taught me that.*

> *Consider it pure joy, my brothers, whenever you face trials of many kinds, because you know that the testing of your faith develops perseverance. Perseverance must finish its work so that you may be mature and complete, not lacking anything.*
>
> —James 1:2–4 NIV

Chapter 44

KIDNEY PUNCH

Chris's routine to get ready for work was like clockwork. Up at 5:15 every morning, he fixed a bowl of cereal and read his Bible at the breakfast table. Next he took his medications and used his prescription inhalers. He watched the news on television while he did his breathing exercises with the incentive spirometer to strengthen his lungs. Then he used an acapella, a plastic device also known as a "pickle" because of its green shape. Blowing into it caused a vibration that loosened mucus in his lungs and helped him cough it up. After that was a nebulizer machine, which changed a liquid saline to a mist that he inhaled into his lungs over a period of twenty minutes. All this took place before he showered and headed out the door by 6:30 or went upstairs to get ready for a conference call.

I found myself grumbling every morning that Chris left his Bible on the kitchen table. *All he has to do is walk five steps to put it back on the end table in the living room where it belongs.* My perspective changed when it dawned on me: *He's working hard to just stay alive. You should be grateful you have a husband who reads his Bible daily and has a job he needs to get ready for.*

Many women aren't so fortunate. Someday that Bible won't be left on the kitchen table ever again, and you'll wish he had left it there.

My attitude changed to gratitude each morning as I put his Bible away for him.

During my morning quiet time with my Bible, I found myself staring at Chris across the room while he read his Bible, savoring that vision. I wanted it imprinted forever in my mind. I knew one day he might no longer be sitting there.

KIDNEY DAMAGE

By January 2016, the cancer battle had taken a tremendous toll on Chris's body. The treatments killed the malignant cells but also damaged his kidneys and other internal structures. He experienced extreme fatigue and slept a lot. Nothing tasted good to him. He prayed that somehow he'd be able to get off the Alimta chemo.

His lab tests showed his creatinine level was double what it should be, so he wasn't able to have chemo at his appointment that week or contrast dye with his scans. He was very anemic and needed a blood transfusion. Chris had so much anxiety thinking about receiving someone else's blood that he vomited before we left home to get the transfusion.

When the nurse took his blood pressure, he tried to do the trick where he elevated his arm to improve the reading because it was very high. The transfusion nurse wouldn't let him. "We need to get a true reading. High blood pressure can cause a stroke and can affect your kidney function."

We hadn't realized he was putting his health at risk by elevating his arm. No one had ever told us high blood pressure affects the kidneys. I was grateful this nurse told us so he wouldn't cheat again.

ARTERITIS

In February, he was referred to a nephrologist (kidney specialist), because his creatinine level was extremely high. Dr. Drummond* said he was between stage 3 and stage 4 of chronic kidney disease (CKD). There are five stages. He explained everything to us in detail and answered all our questions. Chris's condition could be related to kidney stones, high blood pressure, chemo, contrast dye, acid reflux medications, or the use of Excedrin for migraines.

"The damage to your kidneys probably can't be reversed, but we might be able to keep them from getting worse," the doctor said. "We need to avoid kidney toxins and consider the risk-benefit ratio with chemo. I'd like to put chemo on hold, but you need to have a CT scan to make sure we can delay lung cancer treatment."

A kidney biopsy showed Chris had a rare inflammation of the blood vessels called arteritis. It couldn't be prevented or cured, but treatment could help prevent or delay complications. He'd be on steroids for about six months and have to take medications to control their side effects, which included a suppressed immune system. He received an antibiotic to prevent a potentially deadly lung infection called PCP, and he took an antiviral to help prevent chicken pox, shingles, and the flu.

The nephrologist wanted to add rituximab, which is used to treat rheumatoid arthritis and autoimmune disorders. This is a type of chemo, but it's not for lung cancer. The doctor mentioned he would fully support Chris's taking a leave of absence from work during treatment. Chris wasn't ready to do that yet and kept working full time.

If he didn't go back on Alimta, we had only two FDA-approved options available. If it turned out he had an autoimmune disorder, the immunotherapy drug Opdivo would be excluded as an option. Immunotherapy ramps up the autoimmune system to attack cancer. Sometimes it attacks good cells in organs, causing permanent complications. An autoimmune disorder is already ramped up, attacking its own body.

We weren't sure if alectinib would affect his kidneys. Most chemo drugs can potentially affect either the kidney or the liver. He wouldn't qualify for any studies with all his current medical issues.

We were running out of options fast.

> *"Peace I leave with you; My peace I give to you; not as the world gives do I give to you. Do not let your heart be troubled, nor let it be fearful."*
>
> —John 14:27

Chapter 45

WORLD PRAYER

Shane returned on February 24, 2016, from taking care of Chad in Spain. He saw a startling change in his father's condition in the three weeks he was gone and asked if we would be open to the idea of asking for prayer from around the world the next day, seeking immediate healing. Our son's faith and desire to help his dad touched us deeply.

We had been depending on the Lord to put the right doctors and the right medicine in the right place at the right time. Would God show us He didn't need doctors and medicine to do a miracle?

Chris and I sent out a prayer request from Shane to all our family and friends. Our sons contacted their friends too, including those in foreign countries. On February 28, Chris, Shane, and I video chatted with Chad in Spain, and at 1:00 p.m. sharp, we began to pray for Chris's immediate healing. It was a treasured time with family, filled with emotion. The Lord was bombarded with prayers from around the world, including the United States, Canada, Mexico, Colombia, Argentina, Spain, Costa Rica, Brazil, Germany, and the Dominican Republic.

"Again I say to you, that if two of you agree on earth about anything that they may ask, it shall be done for them by My Father who is in heaven. For where two or three have gathered together in My name, I am there in their midst."

—Matthew 18:19–20 NIV

This verse doesn't mean that anything two or more people pray about will be done. It must be prayed for in accordance with *God's* will, not their own. The big question remained, What was God's will for Chris's life?

The next morning, Chris took his medicine as usual. Shane was upset thinking his father didn't trust God to answer the prayers. It wasn't that Chris didn't have faith—there was no proof that God had instantly healed him.

A week later, labs reflected his kidney function was improving. CT scans showed everything was stable, and there was no mention of any suspected tumors. He felt better than he had in the last year. We agreed with the doctors to not restart chemo yet and to let his body continue to recover from the treatments given over the years. Chris enjoyed the break after more than five years of almost constant cancer treatment.

He wrote on CaringBridge:

We seem to be on the right track here and are praying this positive trend continues. Right now, prayer is the best thing we have going. We appreciate all of our prayer warriors!

Hear my prayer, O Lord, listen to my cry for help; be not deaf to my weeping.

—Psalm 39:12 NIV

Chapter 46

WEIGHING TREATMENT OPTIONS

We saw a rheumatologist on March 9. He didn't see any sign of an autoimmune disorder or that the inflammation of the arteries had spread outside the kidneys. That was good news; immunotherapy could still be a possible future cancer treatment option. He thought Chris had renal limited polyarteritis nodosa (PAN), which he didn't think rituximab would help. "No clinical trials have been done with it for your condition. It would be an anecdotal treatment."

I began researching on the internet as soon as we got home and discovered PAN is a serious disease of the blood vessels characterized by damaged arteries that impede the flow of blood to the rest of the body. When the organs don't receive enough blood flow, they have difficulty working and can shut down. Damaged arteries can ultimately affect the heart, brain, and other vital organs, resulting in death from related complications.

We definitely needed prayers.

A week later, we met with Dr. Drummond to go over labs. Chris was still showing improvement, but not enough. He required a more aggressive treatment. The nephrologist, oncologist, and rheumatologist put their heads together and decided to add rituximab chemo—one round per week for four weeks.

I mentioned the rheumatologist had said rituximab was an anecdotal treatment and that no clinical trial had been done to show that it improves PAN.

"Mr. Haga is still alive today because he took chances in the past of unproven treatments," Dr. Drummond pointed out.

The final pathology report from the kidney biopsy showed Chris also had acute interstitial nephritis (AIN), a renal lesion that causes a decline in renal function, usually induced by drug therapy.

In addition to PAN and AIN, he also had necrotizing arteritis and tubular necrosis from decreased blood flow. I felt a surge of panic but tried to keep the terror I felt inside from showing. I didn't understand the condition but knew necrosis meant tissue was dying.

We were given four options, ranging from no treatment (with a poor survival rate) to aggressive treatment. We chose the mildly aggressive treatment of steroids plus rituximab.

I looked through my spreadsheet for treatments Chris had received in the last six years that are known to be hard on the kidneys. In addition to numerous medications, I discovered he had eight PET scans, thirty-six CT scans with contrast, and thirty-nine MRI scans with contrast. No wonder his kidneys weren't happy.

STEROIDS, RITUXIMAB, AND DIETARY RESTRICTIONS

By late March, Chris experienced swelling in his face as well as in his ankles and feet due to the steroids. He didn't look like himself at all. He had to use a diuretic for the swelling and avoid food high in potassium. He also needed to reduce his sodium and protein consumption. He wasn't happy with the dietary restrictions, and it was challenging to find food he liked that he was allowed to eat.

Chris felt good off the chemo. He had a hard time accepting that more chemicals would be dumped into his body to correct a complication that may have been caused by the last chemo. "God's ways are not my ways," he said. "When I prayed to get off Alimta, this is not what I had in mind."

FEELING GOOD

Chris received his first infusion of rituximab on March 28. Less than a week later, he felt great. We went to a movie and to church that weekend. I had trouble keeping up with him in the parking lot, and he wasn't even out of breath. After we got home, he went online and picked out recipes for kidney patients that he was willing to try. Finding those recipes for me took a huge burden off my shoulders while giving him control over what he ate.

During April, Chris cooked meals and helped me with the dishes. He hadn't done that for ages. He even worked in the flower bed. His health was definitely improving.

After seeing his smiling face, I realized the chores made him feel useful again and gave him a sense of accomplishment. It was just what he needed for rejuvenation.

ALECTINIB

After Chris finished his final round of rituximab, Dr. Drummond gave him the okay to be treated again for lung cancer as long as he didn't use Alimta or other drugs toxic to kidneys.

A CT scan on May 9 showed 2 mm spots in the left lung that had grown 1 mm since March.

"We won't be able to find out if they're cancerous because they're too small to biopsy," said Dr. Gerber. "Since you can't have Alimta, it's time to consider starting alectinib."

We discussed the pros and cons of starting it right away. Chris chose to wait and give his kidney function time to improve. He didn't want to be treated for cancer when it wasn't definite the cancer had returned.

SATURATION POINT

In addition to researching drug studies, I had gained valuable input from lung cancer patients with the ALK mutation and their caregivers on inspire.com. I had also joined a Facebook page for "ALKies."

I became overwhelmed with all the correspondence, especially when so few viable options remained for Chris. I had reached my saturation point of acquiring information and desperately needed to escape from the world of cancer. I unsubscribed from the groups and relinquished my co-pilot wings to the Pilot in charge of this epic journey.

I will instruct you and teach you in the way you should go;
I will counsel you and watch over you.

—Psalm 32:8 NIV

Chapter 47

THE BEGINNING OF THE END

In mid-May 2016, I aspirated after a routine procedure and developed pneumonia. While hospitalized, I experienced a bit of Chris's world of many needle pokes. I definitely would rather be the caregiver than the patient.

That evening, I sent Chris home to get my computer and toiletries. When he got back to my hospital room, he sat in the chair, struggling to catch his breath. I was shocked he had such difficulty.

"Are you okay?" I asked.

Unable to speak, he shook his head, blinking back tears. The fright in his eyes scared me. Instead of asking him to spend the night with me in the hospital, I sent him home, where he would get a better night's sleep.

I watched from my window as he trudged to his truck. I'd never seen him walk so slowly. *Lord, please don't let him pass out and fall,* I prayed.

As soon as I was dismissed from the hospital, Chris called Dr. Gerber's nurse. "I'm ready to start alectinib." He took his first dose on May 20.

With cancer, you can give up or you can give it all you've got. Chris made a conscious decision to do the latter for six years. He was willing to get back in the boxing ring one more round, even though the prizefight was taking a tremendous toll on him.

A week later, Chris experienced difficulty while getting ready for work and told me, "I'm out of breath, out of energy, and out of motivation. I don't know why I keep doing what I do." Yet he didn't want to go on disability or retire.

IN CAHOOTS WITH THE NURSE PRACTITIONER

By May 30, Chris was only pulling 1,500 on the incentive spirometer. After taking a shower, he had to sit on the edge of the bathtub to catch his breath. He began sobbing. "I can't even take a shower. I feel like I'm dying. What's the use of living if I can't breathe? I can't do anything."

The next day, I spoke with our friend Starla, a nurse who has the same rare form of lung cancer as Chris and has been on Xalkori (crizotinib) for four years with no evidence of disease as of this writing. Chris was so excited when we met Starla at church in 2014—a beneficiary of his trial.

She asked how Chris was doing.

"I know he's going to need to go on oxygen soon, and he's balking at the suggestion," I replied. "He feels like that would be the beginning of the end. I don't know what to do."

"Call his nurse," she said. "Have her suggest a test to assess his need for oxygen. If she deems it necessary, let her be the one to convince him he needs it. The news will be more acceptable to him if someone with medical authority tells him he needs it instead of coming from his wife. Let him know this may not be a permanent need, but it would help him get through this current bump in the road."

I emailed Sharon, Dr. Gerber's nurse practitioner, and explained the situation. She agreed to the assessment and wouldn't tell Chris I had asked for it.

At his appointment on June 2, for the first time, Chris used a wheelchair offered to him at the valet parking. When Sharon walked into the exam room, she was shocked to see him in it.

"What's this for?" she asked.

"I'm not able to walk far without getting out of breath."

After looking at his vitals, she saw his oxygen at rest was down to 95 percent. "I think it would be a good idea to give you a walking test to see if you need supplemental oxygen."

"I don't want to go on oxygen."

"Would you be willing to at least take a test? The magic number to be concerned about needing supplemental oxygen is 88 percent. Right now, you're at 95 percent."

He consented. A nurse took him for a short walk, and his oxygen went down to 89 percent. "Since that's so close to the magic number, let's test you again, but walk a little farther," Sharon said.

That time his oxygen got down to 85 percent by the time he went halfway. The nurse had to wheel him back to the exam room. Chris still didn't want to use supplemental oxygen.

"I think we should order it for you so you can have it at home if you need it. It's better to have it and not need it than to need it and not have it," Sharon said.

He reluctantly agreed.

I winked and gave her a thumbs-up sign when Chris wasn't looking.

AN UNEXPECTED OUTBURST

Back at home, Chris emailed his supervisor, telling her the doctor was putting him on oxygen, making it challenging to go to the office. She and the occupational nurse agreed to let him work from home for three months, and then they would reevaluate. He was grateful they were willing to let him continue working.

"It makes me feel useful and keeps my mind occupied instead of sitting around all day watching TV and thinking about my problems."

I was relieved to hear that. I still felt guilty for not encouraging him to retire when he was so miserable going to work and wanting to take early retirement. My intuition had told me he would need the work someday just to feel useful.

A few years earlier, Mom had bought a walker with a seat for her future use, thinking Chris might need to borrow it. She also stored my dad's lightweight transport wheelchair for the same reason. Despite Chris's protest, I went to Mom's apartment and brought them both home to have on hand in case he needed them. He wasn't happy with me.

The local durable medical equipment company I found the previous year called about delivering the oxygen supplies to the house. When Chris finished talking with the representative, he gently laid the phone back in the cradle and softly stroked it.

That's odd, I thought.

He suddenly pounded his fist on the filing cabinet next to the fax machine, a gesture totally out of character for him.

"Stop!" I scolded.

"You don't understand—I'm mad as h---!"

What's happening to us? We never yell at each other, and Chris never cusses.

"Are you mad at me?" I asked cautiously.

"No." He choked back tears. "All I have left is food, water, and breath. I pray at night for God to not take those away, and He's now taken my breath away. I have nothing to live for."

BREATHING DIFFICULTIES

On Friday, June 3, he had greater difficulty breathing when walking.

"I'm either going to have to be on oxygen full time or sit in this chair full time."

I suggested we get a shower chair, but he didn't want one, even though he said he wasn't able to stand up long enough to take his shower. I ordered a chair anyway. Then I gave Chris a bath.

"This is humiliating," he said, tears streaming down his face.

I felt so sorry for him. The man of the house—the strong leader of our home—no longer had the capacity to wash himself. He had become unwillingly dependent on me.

How am I going to get him up out of this tub? What if he can't stand up on his own? What if he falls? Panic set in fast. I don't know how we got him to a standing position, but we succeeded. *I never want to do that again. That shower chair had better get here fast.*

Around 11:30 a.m., Chris became concerned because the oxygen still hadn't arrived. The DME company was waiting to get the corrected order from UT Southwestern. "They'd better deliver the oxygen today," he said, "because I don't think I can make it this weekend without it."

In less than twenty-four hours, he went from being mad and not wanting oxygen to realizing he needed it. Even though the DME company didn't have all the proper orders yet, around 4:30 they delivered a home unit and three large E tanks for backup in case of power outage so Chris wouldn't be without oxygen over the weekend. And they didn't charge a penny or require a credit card. Now *that* is good customer service.

DO NOT RESUSCITATE ORDER

Chris had trouble sleeping that night. I got up around 2:00 a.m. to check on him in the living room and encouraged him to come back to bed. When he got there, he was struggling to breathe worse than ever before. We were terrified.

"I'm getting oxygen, but my lungs aren't working," he said.

"If anything happens and you stop breathing, do you want to be resuscitated?"

"No!" he replied without hesitation. "Do *not* bring me back from heaven. That's the only place I will get relief!"

"If you don't want to be resuscitated, you need to sign a DNR [do not resuscitate form] as soon as possible and put it on the refrigerator. I'll also carry a copy of it with us in my binder."

"We can probably get Mary and Zayne [neighbors] to witness it," he said.

"I'll find a form and print it out for you in the morning."

We were talking about his impending death with no emotion. It was all matter-of-fact conversation as if this were nothing out of the ordinary. But we knew this time would eventually come. I then brought up the sensitive subject of his bath.

"It made me sad to know you were humiliated for me to give you a bath. I'm honored to be able to help care for you. You would do the same thing for me—and you have. You helped me bathe after my surgeries. Please let me help you without feeling humiliated. I want to do it because I love you."

"I love you too." He gently kissed me and held me in his arms as we finally drifted off to sleep.

> *My flesh and my heart may fail, but God is the strength of my heart and my portion forever.*
>
> —Psalm 73:26 NIV

Chapter 48

THE BASIC NECESSITIES OF LIFE

Because Chris's creatinine level was way too high again on June 2, he had to stop taking alectinib. On June 8, I found a report on a government website dated May 25, 2016, showing that patients with the ALK mutation have very low overall response rates to Opdivo. This meant the drug was no longer a viable option for Chris because the risk of side effects outweighed any benefit. There were no other new FDA-approved treatments, and Chris wouldn't qualify for clinical trials with his health status.

We were officially out of treatment options.

PLANNING A TRIP TO COLORADO

Chris could now reach only 1,250 on the incentive spirometer. He was too discouraged to ever try it again. We received a G3 Inogen Oxygen Concentrator that he had ordered for trips away from home. The device weighed less than 5 pounds and created its own oxygen supply via a battery.

We started making plans to drive to Colorado and attend Chad and Kate's engagement party on June 18. We were looking forward to meeting Kate's family and friends. We discussed the logistics of the trip. How many portable oxygen tanks should we take with us? Where could we get more if we needed them? We planned to take the large home unit and plug it in at the hotel. I looked up hospital information in case of an emergency. Although the trip wouldn't be easy, Chris wanted to go. Mom tried to discourage us from traveling, afraid we'd be out in the middle of nowhere on the road and need emergency assistance. I worried about that also.

On June 9, Chris's breathing worsened. "Something's not right," he said. "We must be missing something." He asked to get a chest x-ray to see if he had fluid on his lungs. Because he had to keep increasing the oxygen level at home, we also scheduled an appointment with Dr. Gerber for that afternoon.

"The x-ray report shows there's a small basal effusion and possible lymphangitic spread in the left lung. How are you feeling this week?" his doctor asked.

"I feel worse than I did a week ago and worse than just two days ago," Chris said.

"You need to go to the emergency room to see if an intravenous diuretic will help reduce the fluid around your lung. They might have to do a thoracentesis, but I want to try the noninvasive approach first with Lasix. With a thoracentesis, we run the risk of it collapsing the lung."

We discussed going to Colorado the following week.

"I won't authorize you fly. You can drive, but if you feel like this next week, you can't go to Colorado."

Before we left, Dr. Gerber signed the out-of-hospital DNR order.

IN-HOSPITAL DNR ORDER

The following day, Chris had trouble catching his breath in the hospital.

"I know God does things for good, but I don't see any good in this," he said between gasps.

I called the nurse and made sure she knew he had an out-of-hospital DNR order. Since that form is only good outside of a hospital, Chris gave the necessary authorization for the in-hospital DNR. I also made sure the hospital knew he did not want to be intubated.

The nurse turned his oxygen up from level 3 to 4. The diuretic eliminated almost 3 liters of fluid from his body in the first twelve hours. His breathing improved, and so did his state of mind.

RESTRICTIONS

On June 11, we learned that Chris's kidneys were causing the fluid retention. The nephrologist wanted him to continue the IV diuresis. The hospitalist put Chris on a low-sodium diet and limited him to no more than 1 liter of fluid per day from all sources, or roughly four glasses. It was tough to cut back that drastically. He had been used to sipping water all day long while on chemo. He used up a fourth of his allowable intake just taking his medication that morning.

Chris had been praying that God wouldn't take away his breath, food, or water. God wasn't answering those prayers and seemed to be taking away all three.

The hospital computer system is strict when ordering through the kitchen. Unfortunately, the computer didn't realize Chris was unable to eat most of what he had ordered earlier in the day. He ordered a hamburger for supper, but the hospital wouldn't allow him to have ketchup.

"That would put you over your sodium intake allowed."

He didn't want a hamburger without ketchup, so he ordered a flavored ice dessert, which was one item he could keep down.

"That would put you over your fluid intake allowed."

He ordered a salad but didn't like it, so I went to the cafeteria and snuck a hamburger with ketchup into his room. He ate only a portion of the patty, but at least he got some solid food in him before nausea struck.

With the basic necessities of life being taken away, he was losing his will to live.

"Now I urge you to take some food. You need it to survive."
—Acts 27:34 NIV

Chapter 49

SAYING OUR GOOD-BYES

Shane had been in Mexico since April doing missionary work. Chad was still in Europe. We deliberately avoided telling them of their dad's condition. We didn't want them to worry unnecessarily, but the main reason was that Chad was racing. We didn't want to distract his focus.

I was elated to hear from Chad on Friday morning, June 10. He was finished racing for a month and was on his way back to his apartment in Spain. He planned to fly to Dallas on Tuesday before heading on to Colorado for his engagement party.

I finally had the perfect opportunity to fill him in on his dad's condition. "If you fly home earlier than Tuesday, we could spend more time with you," I added. "We may not be able to go to your engagement party."

Chad changed his flight plans and arrived at the hospital Saturday night. When he walked through the door, I hugged him tighter than usual and didn't want to let go. It was the first time I had held my son since he was nearly killed in the head-on collision in January. The scars on his neck still looked fresh and painful. They were a beautiful reminder from God that life is precious and shouldn't be taken for granted.

NURSE NGUYET

Nurse Nguyet gave special attention to Chris and got to know about his personal life and his faith. Before leaving, she asked if the doctors were going to tap his lung with a thoracentesis.

"We're trying to avoid it," I said. "We're afraid it could collapse his only good lung. Are our fears valid?"

The look on her face said she'd rather not answer. She hesitated, then responded, "I would be scared too. It would be best to get this resolved noninvasively. It will be a balancing act to find the right amount of fluids to drink without overloading his lungs yet protecting his kidneys from chemo."

I appreciated her honesty, apparently given from real-life observation.

After her final shift that week, she made a special trip back by Chris's room to tell him good-bye and to pray over us. Overwhelmed with her kindness, Chris and I both grabbed tissues when she left.

SAYING OUR GOOD-BYES

The evening of June 13 was tough emotionally. Long hospital stays have a way of playing havoc with the mind. Chris was pessimistic. He wasn't afraid of death, but he was terrified of prolonged suffering and suffocating while conscious.

"I feel like everything is going downhill. I'm probably going to die from either cancer or kidney problems. The question is, How painful will it be, and how soon?"

I, too, was scared of how he might possibly suffer in the end. Numerous scenarios frequently ran through my mind. None of them occurred. I would have saved myself a lot of heartache if I had remembered there's no need to worry—God's got everything under His control. I'll admit it was easier to worry than to turn to prayer. That's why our prayer warriors were such a necessity to get us through each day.

I climbed into the hospital bed next to Chris. "I've tried to stay strong for you, but I'm crumbling inside right now," I confessed.

We held each other tight as our emotions poured out and he admitted feeling the same. "I'm so tired of fighting the battle. I'm willing to try alectinib again, but I don't think it's going to help. I probably won't even be allowed to take it because of my kidneys."

I remembered my friend Lou Ann's advice from years ago. *There will come a day when Chris says he's had enough and wants to stop treatment. It's his body, and you'll need to be prepared to accept his wishes.* I shared her words of wisdom with him.

"As much as I don't want you to die, I know you're tired, and your quality of life isn't good. When you decide you've had enough, I'll respect your wishes."

We shared how much we loved each other.

I thanked him for being such a wonderful husband, father, and provider. "If I had known before we married that I would be a caregiver to you for six years as you battled lung cancer, and knowing how much I love you now and cherish every second with you, I would've married you all over again in a heartbeat. I'm so grateful that God gave you to me."

Yes, Chris was God's gift to me, but he came with strings attached. And someday God would want him back.

"We'll be together as long as God wishes," I said as tears flowed down our cheeks. "But your love will carry me for my lifetime."

> *Love is patient, love is kind. It does not envy, it does not boast, it is not proud. It is not rude, it is not self-seeking, it is not easily angered, it keeps no record of wrongs. Love does not delight in evil but rejoices with the truth. It always protects, always trusts, always hopes, always perseveres. Love never fails. . . . And now these three remain: faith, hope and love. But the greatest of these is love.*
>
> —1 CORINTHIANS 13:4–8, 13 NIV

Chapter 50

PLANNING AHEAD

It was 1:00 a.m. on June 14. I had been tossing and turning on the couch at the hospital. Mulling over Chris's medical hurdles as well as our conversation, I had a bad feeling in the pit of my stomach. *Things aren't looking promising. I think we need to meet with the funeral home and buy our plots before Chris takes a turn for the worse. We can't put this off any longer.* Although the lights were out, the monitors cast a dim glow in the room. I looked over at my husband. He was sitting up in bed, wide awake, staring off into space.

"I see you can't sleep either," I said. "What are you thinking about?"

"It's time to make funeral arrangements," he said matter-of-factly.

"I was thinking the same thing," I said, strangely calm.

We knew this day would eventually come. We'd been praying for the best for six years. Now it was time to prepare for the worst. I got up, turned on the lights, and sat beside Chris in the hospital bed. I took notes while he started naming off things to do that had been going through his mind.

"Buy our cemetery plots, make sure you're named as beneficiary on everything, tell my boss I'm ready to take a leave of absence from work, and find out about hospice care." He even told me which suit, tie, and belt he wanted to be buried in. We discussed whether I should sell the house or stay in it. He told me who to call if I needed help making financial or other major decisions.

I already carried his medical power of attorney, directive to physicians, and DNR documents with us, and his hospitals had a copy. As soon as we picked out our cemetery plots and made funeral arrangements, he would be "good to go." Since he brought up hospice care, I admitted I had already interviewed two agencies in our insurance network.

"I should've known you'd be prepared for anything."

FLUID DEPRIVATION

The treatment and dietary restrictions were successful in reducing almost all the swelling in Chris's ankles and feet. He lost 12 pounds in just four days between the diuretics and not eating. Doctors had done all they could do for his kidneys, and they dismissed Chris.

At home that evening, he asked for a Popsicle or something to drink.

"You've met your quota already," I said.

"I'm parched and can't even have anything to drink. What's the point in living? God, just take me!" he cried.

The next day, I emailed Dr. Drummond asking if Chris could have more than 1 liter of fluids. He authorized a more realistic 1.5 liters, or 50 ounces.

RETHINKING ENGAGEMENT PARTY AND WEDDING PLANS

We officially cancelled our plans to drive to Colorado for the engagement party. Traveling a long distance, especially to a higher altitude, wouldn't be in Chris's best interest.

Two days before the engagement party, Kate offered to reschedule it so we could attend another time. We nixed that idea. She also offered to scrap the entire wedding plans and start over to hold it in Texas so Chris would be able to attend more easily in October. We rejected that idea also. All the planning and rearranging wouldn't guarantee we'd be able to attend. Realistically, he could be in the hospital, in hospice, or not even be alive by October.

FEET WASHING

By June 18, movement of any kind had become laborious for Chris. He had to sit on an old bar stool at the bathroom sink to shave, resting occasionally to catch his breath. He experienced difficulty breathing when I gave him a shower, even though he had draped the long oxygen hose over the wall. Despite his initial resistance, he now appreciated the shower chair. The exertion of walking three steps from the sink into the shower was almost more than he could handle. Simply leaning his head back while I rinsed his hair wore him out.

I wished I could give him a nice, relaxing, leisurely shower to pamper him, but we didn't have the luxury. It was a race against time. *I have to get him clean and out of this shower before he passes out, or we're going to be in a heap of trouble.* I was praying he wouldn't fall and break the glass.

That morning as I washed his feet, I noticed his toes were turning purple. *He's not getting oxygen to his extremities.* A moment of panic swept over me. I hurriedly finished his feet and turned to tell Chris we were done.

He was crying. "Thank you for being Jesus to me."

I knew Chris appreciated everything I was doing for him, but he didn't say it often. To hear him compare me to Jesus was the sweetest thing he could have said. My heart melted. I loved my husband so much, I would do anything to help him.

"I just wish I had the power to heal you." I gently cupped his face with my hands and kissed him. Tears streamed down my cheeks.

> *Now before the Feast of the Passover, Jesus knowing that His hour had come that He would depart out of this world to the Father, having loved His own who were in the world, He loved them to the end. . . . Then He poured water in the basin, and began to wash the disciples' feet and to wipe them with the towel with which He was girded. . . . So when He had washed their feet, and taken His garments and reclined at the table again, He said to them, "Do you know what I have done to you? You call Me Teacher and Lord; and you are right, for so I am. If I then, the Lord and the Teacher, washed your feet, you also ought to wash one another's feet. For I gave you an example that you also should do as I did to you. Truly, truly, I say to you, a slave is not greater than his master, nor is one who is sent greater than the one who sent him. If you know these things, you are blessed if you do them."*
>
> —John 13:1, 5, 12–17

FATHER'S DAY

On June 19, Father's Day, we video chatted with Chad and Kate in Colorado and Shane in Mexico. Chris was unusually quiet. I could tell he wasn't feeling well. During that night, he complained that his pain was a level 8.

"Jesus, Jesus, Jesus," he whispered softly over and over, trying to summon Him. "Just take me now, Jesus."

I was thankful we didn't attempt the trip to Colorado that weekend.

FUNERAL PREARRANGEMENTS

On Wednesday, June 22, I found Chris sitting on the floor next to his recliner with his head and arms on the seat.

"Why are you on the floor?"

"It's easier to breathe this way."

He had turned his oxygen up to 4.5.

I later found him sitting on Mom's walker in the living room. He had made it from his recliner to the walker across the room, but he needed to rest before walking farther. That was the first time he had used the walker. *Good thing I brought it home, huh?*

Leaving for our appointment at the funeral home, Chris walked five steps before sitting at the kitchen table, gasping. At his request, I turned the oxygen up to level 5. We were scared to death.

"Do you want me to cancel the appointment?"

"No, I want to go do this."

No one wants to make funeral arrangements. He wanted to make sure I wouldn't have to make the decisions by myself. He knew the end was near and was determined to selflessly show his last act of love for me.

Once he caught his breath, I grabbed the wheelchair, and we drove to meet with the funeral director to preplan both our funerals. We were there four hours, filling out the necessary paperwork and picking out caskets, flowers, and a headstone. Before driving to select the cemetery plot, Chris stopped to use the restroom. While waiting for him in the hallway, the director asked about Chris's health.

"At the rate he's going downhill, I wouldn't be surprised if he doesn't make it through the weekend," I whispered softly.

GIVING A HEADS-UP

I vacillated between telling our sons I didn't think their dad would survive much longer and keeping quiet. *Is this "it" or just another temporary setback? Will Chris have another miraculous recovery, or is his time truly nearing the end?* I decided on June 20 to tell the boys so they could make arrangements to spend time with him if they wanted to. I told Shane I might need his muscles soon to help his dad get around. And I asked Chad to release his dad from his promise to be at their wedding.

Shane had planned to leave Mexico on June 24 or June 25 and make the drive over two or three days, but he felt the need to come back sooner. He got out of his two-year missionary commitment, packed all his belongings in his truck, and left Mexico on June 23. He drove twenty-five hours straight through, bringing along his girlfriend for us to meet. He intended to stay as long as necessary to help me with his father.

"Your Father knows what you need before you ask Him."
—Matthew 6:8

Chapter 51

BEGGING

"Jesus, hurry up. Just take me now!" Chris begged.

By June 23, Chris was out of breath just standing. He was ready for the end to come. It was agonizing to watch him struggling, but it also made it easier for me to be willing to let him go. It didn't appear God intended to heal him this time. He couldn't ride his bike, do photography, eat, sleep, or work. He didn't even have the stamina to stand up. His food, water, and breathing were restricted. He had absolutely no pleasures or quality of life left.

"I feel like God has abandoned me. Why isn't He answering?" asked Chris.

It finally dawned on me. "Everyone is praying for you to live, but we're praying now for God to take you. We need to pray for God's will and His timing and ask others to do the same."

As the morning progressed, Chris struggled to breathe, so we raised his oxygen level to 5.5, the highest it could go on the tank at home.

"I think we need to go to the ER," I said.

"I don't want to go to the ER again."

"At least let me call UT Southwestern."

"Okay," he relented.

The nurse told me to take him to their Richardson location, which was about twenty minutes from home. If needed, they would take him to the hospital by ambulance.

Chris grabbed the portable oxygen concentrator and the backup battery pack. I got our prepacked suitcases and the lightweight transport wheelchair. I tried to wheel Chris over the threshold to the garage but couldn't get over it. He stood up so I could get the wheelchair out the door. That left him breathless. Pushing him to the car, I almost tipped him over as we went down a small cement lip from the garage to the driveway. Once inside the car, his struggle to breathe was worse than ever. Chris sobbed. All this was more than he could handle.

"Do you want me to call an ambulance?" I asked.

"No, they'll just take me to the nearest hospital. Get in and take me to UT Southwestern."

He calmed down once we got underway. We drove in silence, deep in our own thoughts. I was too scared to talk or ask questions. I was afraid of the answers.

In the waiting room at the clinic, Chris stared at the television while I checked messages on my phone. I found a Facebook message from Ben Kendall, a family friend who had lived with us years earlier while he was in seminary. I am sharing with his permission.

He wrote, "I read the post about Shane coming home. I know that wouldn't happen unless things were getting pretty bad. I'm so sorry, and I will be continuing to lift you and Chris up. I pray that your love strengthens with each moment. Never forget that God is always with you and He feels your pain with you. He does not distance Himself and He embraces you when you are overwhelmed. He satisfies you when you feel empty and hopeless. He can take your anger when you are mad or frustrated. He will be your listener when you just need to spill your emotions out. He will uphold you when you feel like it is going to fall apart.

May God pour out the same love, compassion, and mercy that matches and even supersedes the anguish you must be feeling."

"Thank you. Chris feels God has abandoned him," I answered hastily.

"Then I will pray for God to reveal Himself. You are being Christ to him. God has a reason. This has not been in vain. Many people have been encouraged by your faith through the last few years. Many people have been changed for the better. What Satan has meant for evil, God has made good."

"He's been crying out to God to take him. He is miserable, and it's so scary when he's gasping for air," I responded.

"Are you ready for God to take him? As much as you could be?" Ben asked.

"YES," I replied emphatically.

"I'm feeling that on this end. I'll pray for relief. You're an amazing person. I mean that from the bottom of my heart. Chris has been blessed to have you as his wife. God chose you to be his soul mate, and you are the only one who could have been fashioned for him to go through this with. Please let Chris know I'm praying and that God has made me a better person because of his testimony."

"Thank you for your prayers for us."

I handed my phone to Chris and shared the messages. After he silently handed the phone back, I hoped he didn't think I was eager for him to die when I typed, "YES." I was only saying I was ready to let him go if that was God's plan.

"Yes. It is well with my soul," is what I wanted to type. I'm fast on a keyboard with two hands, but I'm slow at texting on my phone with one finger. We were the only ones left in the waiting room, and I was trying to finish my conversation with Ben before we got called to see the nurse.

When the nurse examined Chris, his oxygen saturation was 87 percent.

"You need to go to the hospital. I can either call an ambulance, or you can ride in your car. If you go in an ambulance, they won't take you to Clements Hospital—they will take you to the nearest one."

Chris said, "We made it here in the car okay, so I'll just go in the car. I only want to go to Clements."

Under proper medical attention at the hospital, Chris relaxed, his vitals improved, and he felt better. Scans showed the fluid in his lungs was unchanged from his last hospital stay; he didn't want them to drain it.

Chad and Kate arrived from Colorado at 10:00 p.m. After they left, Chris complained of back discomfort. His pain level rose to an 8 despite having received hydrocodone. He called the nurse, begging for morphine. He asked for 8 mg, since he had been prescribed 15 mg before for back pain after surgery several years previously. Half of a dose had helped well enough before, so he assumed he could have a similar dosage and it would have the same effect again.

The night-shift doctor only let him have 1 mg of morphine. *It's going to be a rough night,* I thought.

> *Therefore we do not lose heart. Though outwardly we are wasting away, yet inwardly we are being renewed day by day. For our light and momentary troubles are achieving for us an eternal glory that far outweighs them all. So we fix our eyes not on what is seen, but on what is unseen. For what is seen is temporary, but what is unseen is eternal.*
>
> —2 Corinthians 4:16–18 NIV

Chapter 52

IT IS WELL

The morning of June 24, Chris couldn't get comfortable at all. He moved back and forth from the bed to the chair several times during the night, trying to find a position to relieve his back pain. I couldn't sleep either. I was afraid he would pass out while walking or trip over his oxygen hose or the IV stand.

Around 1:00 a.m., he asked for hydrocodone for his pain, which had greatly improved after the morphine earlier. Three hours later he was in misery again, so he asked for morphine.

The nurse said, "The doctor doesn't like to prescribe it without the primary care doctor's knowledge. We can give you hydrocodone again."

Chris adamantly refused the hydrocodone. "It. Doesn't. Help. I need *morphine*!"

The night-shift nurse then paged the on-call doctor, but he would only give a one-time order for 1 mg of morphine.

By 8:00 that morning, Chris and I were already exhausted. We'd had only one hour's sleep all night. He rated his pain level a 10 by the time the doctor with the authority stopped by to see him.

"I'll authorize four milligrams of morphine. If that's not enough, I'll authorize more, but I don't want to start with eight milligrams." He turned to me. "Someone has to be in the room with him at all times in case he has a bad reaction."

I assumed he was talking about an allergic reaction like my dad had to a medication in the hospital. I had no reason to think otherwise.

The doctor wanted to do an ultrasound of the abdomen, thinking a tumor might be pressing on a nerve and causing the pain. After injecting the morphine intravenously, the nurse put Chris on a higher-flow oxygen tube at level 6.

"Do you want me to ask Taylor to come pray with us?" I asked Chris. Taylor Gardner was the pastor from our church Care Ministry and led the Cancer Encouragement Group.

"Yes. But I don't want to see anyone else today outside of family. I just don't feel up to it."

An hour later, Chris received another 2 mg of morphine. His pain level decreased from 10 to 4. But his breathing was worse.

RAPID RESPONSE TEAM

Shane called around 10:00 a.m. while Chris was getting the ultrasound. He and his girlfriend were in Tucson, Arizona, which was still a long way from Dallas. I told him his dad wasn't doing well and was going downhill fast.

"Prepare for the possibility he might not be here when you arrive."

During the sonogram, they had to bump Chris's oxygen up to level 9. He looked like death warmed over when he got back to the room and had a hard time breathing. I couldn't believe how bad he looked compared to just forty-five minutes earlier.

When I found out how much oxygen they were giving him, I silently freaked out. *His portable oxygen concentrator and the oxygen tank at home only go up to 5.5. How are they going to get him back down to that level so he can go home?*

I texted Chad and Kate, "Can you come soon?"

Chad called me immediately. "Do I sense an urgency because you didn't ask, '*When* are you coming?' "

"Yes. He's not doing well at all."

"Okay, we'll be there as soon as we can."

I handed my phone to Chris so he and Chad could talk. Chad told me later he didn't recognize his dad's voice. They said their I love yous in case that was the last time they spoke.

Numerous "white coats" and nurses suddenly appeared in the room. It was standing room only. I didn't comprehend what was happening. I found out two months later from reading the medical reports that this was a rapid response team (RRT) that had been summoned, plus probably fellows or interns.

Then Taylor arrived. He hesitated, not knowing whether to come in or wait.

I motioned him in.

A nurse put an oxygen mask on Chris. After about thirty seconds, he panicked. "Take it off. It's making me claustrophobic."

The hospital oncologist talked with him. "Lasix didn't help your breathing. There was no infection seen on the x-rays. Either cancer or a pleural effusion has damaged your lung. The increase in oxygen hasn't worked. We can't do chemotherapy because of your kidney function. We can't do surgery because of your health. The only option left is a thoracentesis to drain five hundred to eight hundred milliliters from the left lung."

Chris nodded. "I'll do the thoracentesis."

I was dumbfounded. We had talked about this several times before, and he had told me, "I don't want to take a risk of collapsing my only good lung."

Thoughts flashed through my mind. *He's been through so much already. Does he remember how painful the thoracentesis is? If his lung collapses during the procedure, that's probably a horrible death of conscious suffocation. I can't let him die alone on the table like that. Shane won't get here until late tonight. He can't die before Shane gets here!*

"Will the thoracentesis help him get well?" I asked the doctor.

"It's unlikely we'll see dramatic improvement."

I knew Chris didn't have the physical strength to fight and had lost his will to live. "Chris, are you sure you want to do the thoracentesis?" I asked. "You almost passed out twice when you had it done before because of the pain. Shane is on his way."

He understood what I left unsaid. Without hesitation, he changed his mind. "I don't want to do the thoracentesis. Just make me comfortable."

"Are you sure? Do you realize what this means?" the doctor asked, looking at both of us.

"Yes," Chris answered.

I nodded. "He's been begging God to take him for the last few weeks." I added, "You do have in your records, don't you, that he signed an in-hospital DNR? And he doesn't want to be intubated."

"Yes, that's in our records. Would you like for me to call a clergy?" the doctor asked.

"No, this is our pastor," I said, pointing toward Taylor.

The doctor hadn't indicated if we were looking at hours, days, weeks, or months. Questioning us about clergy should have clued me in.

Just then, a respiratory therapist came with a BiPAP breathing mask, trying to squeeze through the crowd. Before she could get close to Chris, the doctor shook his head, indicating she shouldn't put it on the patient. She looked at the doctor, puzzled.

"He just wants to be made comfortable at this time," the oncologist said.

The shocked look in her eyes was telling, as if she were thinking, *He will likely die without this.* She quietly gathered her equipment and backed out of the room, followed by the rest of the medical team.

Taylor and I walked over to Chris's bedside, and Taylor prayed for us.

"I want you to do my service," Chris said. "And be sure to share the gospel. There will be people there who need to hear it."

Chris and I were unbelievably calm in the face of death. We had peace even though our life was in turmoil.

FAMILY AND FRIEND TIME

Chad and Kate arrived shortly before noon, and I filled them in on what had taken place since they had left the night before. The morphine was relaxing Chris and making him sleepy. I knew he was tired and needed to rest, so we didn't talk much.

Randy, Molly, and their daughters came to stay with us.

About 1:00 p.m., Shane called again to check on his dad.

"Let Shane talk to Daddy," Chad said.

"But he's driving," I responded.

"You've *got* to let him talk to Daddy!" Chad pleaded. He was afraid Shane might not get to the hospital in time.

"Hey, dude," Chris said when I handed him the phone. His speech was becoming slurred, and he sounded intoxicated. They talked briefly.

Shane did most of the talking. He journaled later in his *Shane Meets World* blog entry "The Cancer Filter."

> *I tried to say everything I could think of, everything I might have left unsaid over the years, yet the doubt in my mind lingered that he wasn't "there" enough to understand.*

"I love you. Drive carefully," Chris said. His mind was still coherent. He understood every word.

He began sweating, so I wiped him down with a cold wash cloth. Several minutes later, I asked him, "Are you still hot?"

"Oh, yeah, baby." He smiled provocatively. He would have winked, but his eyes were closed. He was still able to make everyone in the room laugh.

A little later, I again asked if he was still hot.

He touched his finger to his leg. "*Tssss.*" He was sizzling, causing us to laugh some more.

At one point, Chris had been quiet for a while, napping. Out of nowhere, he looked at Chad and did a Three Stooges move, putting his thumb between his eyes, wiggling his fingers, and saying, "Wa-wa-wa-wa!" in a silly voice. He was trying to lighten the mood by letting us know he was still with us.

Later, Chad and Kate were holding Chris's left hand. Chris reached with his right hand and clasped their hands in his. He spoke with a drug-induced stupor. "Bless you two. Make *lots* and *lots* of babies."

Those are the last words I heard him speak.

He closed his eyes to nap again, found a comfortable position, and completely relaxed. He quickly fell into unconsciousness and developed "the death rattle," a sound similar to snoring that occurs when air passes through the mucus in the throat. The nurse put a scopolamine patch behind his ear to dry the throat secretions. This worked quite well. I was relieved we didn't have to listen to that sound.

Although Chris had told me he didn't want visitors other than family because he didn't feel well, I didn't think that request applied any longer. I remembered how our friend Heather let us visit her husband a few days before he died of lung cancer. She gave us the opportunity to tell him good-bye and get closure. How gracious she was to share her last few days with him so Brett would know how much he was loved by his friends. I wanted that for Chris.

Late that afternoon, I left the room and started calling his closest friends. "I don't want you to feel obligated, but if you want to come say good-bye, I don't want to deny you that opportunity."

I then told my family I desperately needed to close my eyes for a bit but to come get me in the waiting room down the hall if anything happened. I found the quietest spot I could. It felt good to close my eyes, but my mind wouldn't shut off.

Stay alert, DeLayne. You need to remember every moment of today, because these will be your final memories with Chris.

Ten minutes later, I called Chris's supervisor and left a voice message to give her a heads-up that he wouldn't be returning to work so she could keep things running smoothly. Then I returned to be with Chris.

The nurse startled me when she turned the monitors off around 6:30 that evening. Then I remembered when Dad was in the hospital nearing death. I had panicked when some numbers went too low and ran to get Dad's nurse. She had calmly explained he was in palliative care, and things were just taking a natural course as his body was shutting down.

I realized Chris's nurse was trying to prevent distress for the family.

Friends and family arrived throughout the evening to show Chris their love. I had seen Nurse Nguyet in the hospital that morning and told her we were back. She stopped to visit after her shift and was shocked to see Chris in a coma. She began crying and hugged me. In the short time she took care of Chris, she had grown fond of him. I introduced her to the family and told them how good she had been to Chris. This sweet nurse prayed for us before she left.

HOSPICE

Around 7:30 p.m., the nurse told me they would contact hospice.

"I've already picked out a hospice care that's in our insurance network," I said and gave her the information I carried in my notebook.

"We'll call them for you. They will probably contact you in the morning. In the meantime, we will provide hospice care here."

How are we going to get him home for hospice care? By ambulance? Could he survive the trip? I mentally rearranged the furniture in our bedroom to accommodate a hospital bed.

The nurse observed Chris. His respirations were between five and eight per minute.

"How long do you think he has?" I asked.

"He may pass tonight."

"Shane should be here in a little bit, Chris. Hang in there," I said.

VIGIL

Shane and his girlfriend finally arrived at 11:00 p.m. Randy and Molly met them at the elevator to prepare them for what they were about to see. After Shane introduced his girlfriend to everyone, Chad suggested we give Shane some alone time with his dad. My heart ached for him. I knew he was devastated.

Looking at the clock as each minute dragged on, my mind wandered to a dark place. *What will be Chris's date of death?* I couldn't think of any date that had special meaning that he might be hanging on for. Yet he lingered. Everyone was tired and went home at midnight except for the boys, their ladies, and me.

Time ticked on. We kept a vigil around Chris's bed, holding his hands.

"Come on, Chris, we're so tired. What are you waiting for?" I asked. It sounded callous, and my words shocked everyone, including myself. Exhaustion had taken over.

We decided to take shifts watching him. The boys and their sweethearts sat on the small sofa, heads propped against each other, sleeping as best they could as I took the first shift.

Looking over at them asleep, I suddenly felt all alone in the dark room. But I wasn't. A small, quivering smile crept onto my face. *Thank you, Lord, that both boys have their loved one here to comfort them tonight. Thank You for being here for me. I couldn't do this without Your love carrying me through these darkest moments.* Tears of both joy and sorrow flowed down my face as I realized Jesus would be taking the place of my husband.

An hour later, Chris's respirations became extremely shallow, and he was breathing only four times per minute. I tried to match my breathing to his but couldn't even come close. *How is he still alive? His heart must be really strong.*

I stroked his soft, thick hair a lot and kissed his forehead. My love for him deepened as I realized how his example of faith in adversity had refined my own relationship with the Lord these last six years. What a priceless gift that was to me. Chris could have blamed God and walked away from his faith, but he embraced it instead.

Although we had said our good-byes a couple of weeks before, I again whispered in his ear my final farewell. "Thank you for being such a great husband, father, and provider. I couldn't have asked for anyone better. Thank you for loving me. I love you, and I thank God for you. I'm going to miss you, but I'll be okay. I promise."

"I love you, and I thank God for you" were words our minister suggested, during our premarital counseling thirty-two years earlier, to always remember to say to each other.

I found myself nodding off by Chris's bedside, holding his hand. I hadn't slept more than an hour in two nights, and it was catching up with me.

THE PERFECT DEATH SCENE

Over the past six years, I had time to imagine the perfect death scene. In it, Chris was at home in bed with me lying by his side, holding one hand with my other arm draped over his chest in a hug. He would die peacefully in his sleep, knowing he was loved to his last breath. In my scenario, I didn't think the boys would be able to make it home in time.

Simply holding his hand wasn't good enough for me. The boys were cuddled up with their ladies. I wanted to snuggle with my husband. *If I'm asleep when he passes, I want to be holding him in my arms.* I crawled into the hospital bed, squeezing in on his left side between him and the bedrail.

Just as I had imagined, I held Chris's left hand in my right. His hand was growing colder as his body continued to shut down. With my left arm draped over his chest, I watched carefully to make sure I wasn't hindering his breathing. He didn't appear to be in any distress. I closed my eyes and let the sleep come.

At 6:00 a.m., I felt a pressure on my left arm and right hand. I opened my eyes and noticed the sun peeking through the window. The pressure I felt was Chad. He was holding his hand over mine and his father's, resting his head on my arm, and crying. I don't know how long he had been there. Kate was sitting behind him. Shane and his girlfriend were on the other side, with Shane holding his dad's right hand.

I moved enough to put my arm around Chad. We stayed that way for a long time, watching Chris breathe.

"His breathing is changing," Chad said.

The death rattle was back. His breathing was faster but more shallow.

We watched his every breath closely. The nurse checked on him five minutes before her shift ended. When I told her his breathing was rattling again, she left to get another patch to put behind his ear to dry the secretions.

While she was gone, Chad announced, "His breathing is changing again."

Slowly Chris's chest stopped rising up and down. We saw the air making its way up his throat with each final respiration. Then his breathing quietly stopped. I looked at the clock. The second hand rolled over the twelve. It was exactly 7:00 a.m. on

Saturday, June 25, 2016. Chris was finally at peace. He died in a scenario more perfect than I had imagined. Both our sons were with him as he took his final breath.

Assured of Chris's salvation and that he was now with the Lord, I was also at peace in my heart. He faced death courageously, knowing he would soon be spending eternity in heaven. He fought for his life to the end. Although it wasn't the healing on earth that we prayed for, he kept his faith.

> *I have fought the good fight, I have finished the race, I have kept the faith.*
>
> —2 Timothy 4:7 NIV

We were all calmly moving away from the bed when the nurse came in with the medication. I don't think any of us were crying. She looked confused.

"It's over," I said. "He passed away at exactly seven o'clock."

Shane and his girlfriend headed for the house to get some sleep after their twenty-five-hour drive straight through from Mexico, while Chad and Kate waited with me for the doctor and mortician.

The doctor arrived within the hour.

I asked him a question that had been puzzling me. "What happened that caused such a sudden decline in his health yesterday?"

"Probably giving him morphine. It suppresses the respiratory system, and his lungs were already compromised."

I wish we had been told that before he took it. Not that it would have changed Chris's decision to take the medication. It allowed him to die peacefully, painlessly, and fairly quickly, the way he would have wanted. But if we knew that death could come quickly, it would have given us an idea of what to expect so we could say our final good-byes before he went into a coma.

Whenever Chris was in the hospital, the nurse would always write a goal for the day on the whiteboard. Sometimes it was simply "Go home." Before we left the hospital, I grabbed the marker and wrote, "Went home with the Lord." Then I drew a smiley face.

I wanted the medical staff to know, "It is well with my soul."

And the peace of God, which transcends all understanding, will guard your hearts and your minds in Christ Jesus.
—Philippians 4:7 NIV

Chapter 53

THE RIDE OF HIS LIFE

A year before Chris died, he wrote a blog entry that he asked me to post after he died. I had read it then but hadn't looked at it since. This particular entry was so important to him that it was first on his list of things for me to do after his death.

Several hours after he had passed, I started to read through the entry before posting it. I made it through the first two sentences. Running into the kitchen, I asked Chad and Shane, "What time did Daddy usually go on his Saturday morning bike rides?" They could hear the sense of urgency in my voice.

"He usually liked to be out the door by seven o'clock," Chad responded. "Why?"

Tearing up, I realized *that's* what Chris was waiting for—his 7:00 a.m. ride. And what a ride of his life to heaven it must have been on that cool, beautiful June morning.

A Good Ride

Saturday morning was always my favorite time to go for a bike ride. I'd be up, dressed, and out the door before the first rays of sunshine began to peek over the horizon. There was just something about feeling the cool morning breeze on my face and pushing the pedals as the sun rose. Those mornings contain some of my favorite memories. I can remember where I was the first time I rode over thirty miles. The same for when I broke through the fifty-mile-ride limit. The first forty-five miles of that ride were a lot of fun. There was just something about pushing my body a little bit further than I thought it would go. On those mornings, as I rode home, I knew I'd had a good ride.

In many ways, this quest to beat lung cancer has been much the same. Many times I just had to push my body a little bit further than I thought it could go. The times I thought I couldn't make it any further, friends and family would lift us up. Sometimes they would come in person. Sometimes it was in their prayers. I've lost count of the times that DeLayne, the boys, and I have been blessed by the giving of others. Perhaps, the most surprising thing has been the many times we've been blessed by opportunities to give to other people. It's been a long journey that wouldn't have been possible without the help of others and the grace of God.

Yes, this journey has been a long one. There were twists and turns, never knowing what lay beyond the next bend in the road, but learning to trust that Jesus would be there waiting on us. It has taken us places we never thought we'd have to go, both physically and spiritually.

My earthly journey has come to an end. I now know what lay beyond the last bend in the road. I'm finally home resting in the loving arms of my Savior, Jesus Christ.

I've had a good ride.

My frame was not hidden from You, when I was made in secret, and skillfully wrought in the depths of the earth; Your eyes have seen my unformed substance; and in Your book were all written the days that were ordained for me, when as yet there was not one of them.

—Psalm 139:15–16

Chapter 54

DO NOT WORRY

"You worry too much." How many times had I heard that from Chris over the years?

Almost three weeks after Chris passed away, Shane mentioned he planned to make a leather wallet for himself, the craft his dad had taught him. Later, when I went upstairs to tell him good night, he was working on the design. In the bottom right corner, he had drawn a fancy 6 and a 25 with room for two more numbers.

"Thirty-four?" I asked.

"No—sixteen."

In memory of his dad, he was including the date of his dad's death on June 25, 2016.

Confused, he asked, "What made you think it would be the number thirty-four?"

"Matthew 6:25–34 was your dad's all-time favorite scripture. He asked that it be read at his funeral."

It was no accident I had walked in at that exact moment. Sometimes my thought processes are a little slow. It wasn't until the next morning I made the connection between June 25, the day Chris died, and his favorite Bible passage.

I hadn't understood why God prolonged the last day of Chris's life. God had a plan for His timetable. It wasn't a coincidence that Chris passed on Saturday, 6/25, at exactly 7:00 a.m. God knew all along that nothing else would give me such peace about my husband's passing as that date and precise time.

Even through his death, Chris was still reminding me, "Do not worry. God is in control."

> *"For this reason I say to you, do not be worried about your life, as to what you will eat or what you will drink; nor for your body, as to what you will put on. Is not life more than food, and the body more than clothing? Look at the birds of the air, that they do not sow, nor reap nor gather into barns, and yet your heavenly Father feeds them. Are you not worth much more than they? And who of you by being worried can add a single hour to his life? And why are you worried about clothing? Observe how the lilies of the field grow; they do not toil nor do they spin, yet I say to you that not even Solomon in all his glory clothed himself like one of these. But if God so clothes the grass of the field, which is alive today and tomorrow is thrown into the furnace, will He not much more clothe you? You of little faith! Do not worry then, saying, 'What will we eat?' or 'What will we drink?' or 'What will we wear for clothing?' For the Gentiles eagerly seek all these things; for your heavenly Father knows that you need all these things. But seek first His kingdom and His righteousness, and all these things will be added to you.*
>
> *"So do not worry about tomorrow; for tomorrow will care for itself. Each day has enough trouble of its own."*
>
> —Matthew 6:25–34

Chapter 55

HIS LOVE CARRIES ME

When Chris and I visited the Hawaiian island of Kauai, our trip to Waimea Canyon was one of our favorite memories. Of the two routes we could take to the top, we chose the more scenic route, which skirted the canyon rim. On this narrow road we experienced sharp inclines followed by quick descents, switchbacks, and blind curves. I've never done well on roads like these, and I was terrified we would drive off the edge or a car might cross the line coming around a sharp turn. I held Chris's water bottle during the ride. Apparently, I white-knuckled it, since it was crushed when I handed it to him. We never found out if the road was scenic. I couldn't look, and I wouldn't allow him to look, admonishing him multiple times, "Just watch the road."

Despite the agony of the drive, it was worth it. Once we got to the top, the view at Wai'ale'ale was magnificent with lush, green mountain foliage, beautiful white fluffy clouds, and an ocean the same blue color as the sky. You couldn't tell where the sea ended and the sky began. To top it off, there was a rainbow—a sign of God's love and a promise of hope for our future in the present and in eternity. We stood there a long time, soaking in this manifestation of God's creation.

Chris's blog post "What a View" compared our Waimea Canyon excursion to life:

This trip makes me realize that someday we will come to the end of the road on this journey. We'll look back down the road we've been on and see all of the steep climbs, rapid descents, blind corners, and hairpin turns. We'll see all that God has done and His handiwork in our lives.

We will say, "What a view!"

Hawaii has its own native language. Most people know that "aloha" means both "good-bye" and "hello." Some say its literal meaning is "presence of breath" or "the breath of life." The real meaning to Hawaiians is living with the spirit of "love, peace, and compassion"—the kind that endures through all life's tribulations.

Although Chris's odyssey on earth came to an end, that wasn't the end of his life. When God writes His child's story, what appears to be the ending to us is merely the prelude to a new beginning.

In 2011, Chris talked about this in "A Life Sentence."

What has helped me the most is that I don't see cancer as a death sentence. I see it as a life sentence. I firmly believe that God's will is for me to be completely healed from cancer and that it will never return. When that happens, I will live every day with gratitude for that momentous event, loving my family, enjoying the days with them, and I will continue to worship Jesus.

There are some people who will ask, "What if God's will is for you not to be healed?"

If the time should come that cancer takes my earthly body, I am certain that my belief in Jesus Christ means that when I take my last breath on earth, I will then take my first breath in heaven. I will then have two good lungs, and there will be no more pain. I will see my family and friends who have gone before me, and I will continue to worship Jesus.

Either way, I still live!

Because Christ loved us so much, He died on the cross for the forgiveness of our sins. I've accepted Jesus as my personal Savior, so I also have the assurance of spending eternity in heaven when I die.

Christ's love, as well as my husband's, carries me through each day and will continue to do so until I reach my final destiny. I know without a doubt they are both waiting for me in heaven with open arms. When I get there, I will forever experience love, peace, and compassion as never before.

Aloha.

"For God so loved the world, that He gave His only begotten Son, that whoever believes in Him shall not perish, but have eternal life."

—John 3:16

EPILOGUE

We had asked God for a miracle cure. He gave it to us three times. Since it wasn't His will to heal Chris a fourth time, I need to be content with the path chosen for us. I could allow myself to succumb to anger and self-pity, wallowing in my grief. But I refuse to let cancer have the last word in my life. I made a promise to Chris on his deathbed, "I'll be okay." So I'm choosing to have joy in the time I have left here on earth and follow a path of happiness by helping others in a way that both honors my husband's memory and reflects Christ's love.

> *"You will grieve, but your grief will turn to joy."*
>
> —John 16:20 NIV

I miss Chris very much. But I have peace because I can see the bigger picture, especially after writing about our journey through cancer.

HUGE MIRACLE REVEALED

In August 2017, I went to the Dallas Christian Writers Guild monthly meeting, where writers critique each other's work. I almost didn't go because I didn't have anything new ready for critique. I decided to take the revised introduction of my book. Earlier that morning, I had added the fact that Chris's lung tumor had grown to 13 cm before effective treatment was found.

One of the group's members is a retired surgeon who had worked in a trauma unit.

"Most people won't understand the significance of what a tumor that size means, but I do," he said. He began talking about a bell-shaped curve of statistics.

"What does that mean?" I asked.

"The chance of his surviving more than six months with a mass that size was zero percent. It's only because of you, his doctors, and God that he survived six years."

No one had ever given us that statistic before. It wasn't just a small miracle that Chris lived six years. It was a huge miracle that he lived more than six months.

The magnitude of what God did and allowed us to be a part of sank in and overwhelmed me during the middle of that night. Every time I walked across the room for more tissues, my legs were wobbly. I dropped to my knees, sobbing. I bowed in reverence to God for His awesome power to heal and for allowing me to play a role as Chris's caregiver. I finally fully understood what compelled me to write this book. God wanted me to share His love story.

THE LAST WORD

Cancer didn't have the last word—God did. As our friend Tom Wohlgamuth said at the graveside service, "Chris didn't lose his battle with cancer. Cancer lost its battle with Chris. When the cancer conquered his body, the cancer stopped living. It died. Forever. But Chris lives because Jesus conquered sin and death for us!"

Chris gained victory over death. His spirit lives on and continues to help others in their battle and in their walk with the Lord as we share our story with you. I believe this verse answers my husband's long-sought-after purpose for having cancer:

"This sickness will not end in death. No, it is for God's glory so that God's Son may be glorified through it."

—John 11:4 NIV

After Chris was diagnosed with this terminal disease, we spent plenty of time in waiting rooms and hospitals with opportunities to think about the hand we'd been dealt. Cancer reminded us that life is precious, while giving us an opportunity to see God in many different ways.

Although we'll never know exactly why God allowed Chris to have lung cancer, we were blessed to have experienced such an ordeal together. As trite and inconceivable as that might sound, it's true. Our love for each other grew stronger. We learned to not take life or each other for granted. Each day became more treasured as God's hand was revealed, even in difficult moments. We met so many wonderful people we would have never met otherwise.

Our suffering allowed us to experience personal growth. We walked through the fiery furnace and survived, year after year. We emerged with more confidence to face whatever challenges life presented, trusting the Lord was with us. We encouraged others because we'd been down the same path they were on. We tried to be a bright spot in the day for medical professionals who normally saw their patients losing their battles.

Looking back, I see that the struggles and challenges we faced developed our perseverance, character, and hope much better than anything else ever had.

And we rejoice in the hope of the glory of God. Not only so, but we also rejoice in our sufferings, because we know that suffering produces perseverance; perseverance, character; and character, hope.

—Romans 5:2–4 NIV

Best of all, our relationship with the Lord deepened as we felt the depth of His outpouring love for us over and over again. We realized that even if Chris were to lose his battle against the cancer, we could find comfort knowing he would still have eternal life with the Lord. What greater love is there?

God deeply loves you. You don't believe it? Look at the cross. He loved His Son yet sacrificed Him to pay the penalty for our sins so that we would be able to spend eternity in heaven.

You may not have cancer, but your life is terminal. You just don't necessarily know what your cause of death will be or when your time will be up. Do you know, without a doubt, where you will spend eternity if you were to die today?

Have you accepted His love or rejected it? Can you imagine being a parent and having your child reject your love and shut you out of his life? Your grief wouldn't compare to the grief our heavenly Father must feel if you reject His free gift of eternal salvation.

"But I've lived a life full of sin. How could God love me?" you may ask.

There's no sin so big He won't forgive you. Denying Christ is the only thing that will prevent you from entering the kingdom of heaven. If you've never invited Jesus into your life but want to do so, simply pray something like this:

> *"Dear Lord, I admit I've sinned in my life and ask you to forgive me. I believe You're the Son of God and that You died on the cross to take the punishment for my sin. I believe You were buried and rose again from the grave. Thank You for Your gift of eternal life. I accept that gift and invite you into my life as my personal Savior. I choose to follow You into eternity. It's in Jesus' name I pray. Amen."*

> *For the wages of sin is death, but the free gift of God is eternal life in Christ Jesus our Lord.*
>
> —Romans 6:23

Appendix A

LUNG CANCER STATISTICS AND SYMPTOMS

- Ten to fifteen percent of lung cancer cases are in never-smokers.
- Sixty to sixty-five percent of all new lung cancer diagnoses are among people who have never smoked or are former smokers.[1]

The signs and symptoms of lung cancer can take years to develop, and they may not appear until the disease is advanced. Some symptoms of lung cancer are in the chest:

- Coughing, especially if it persists or becomes intense
- Pain in the chest, shoulder, or back unrelated to pain from coughing
- A change in color or volume of sputum
- Shortness of breath
- Changes in the voice or being hoarse
- Harsh sounds with each breath
- Recurrent lung problems, such as bronchitis or pneumonia

- Coughing up phlegm or mucus, especially if it is tinged with blood
- Coughing up blood

If the original lung cancer has spread, a person may feel symptoms in other places in the body. Common places for lung cancer to spread include other parts of the lungs, lymph nodes, bones, brain, liver, and adrenal glands. Some symptoms of lung cancer that may occur elsewhere in the body:

- Loss of appetite or unexplained weight loss
- Muscle wasting
- Fatigue
- Headaches, bone or joint pain
- Bone fractures not related to accidental injury
- Neurological symptoms, such as unsteady gait or memory loss
- Neck or facial swelling
- General weakness
- Bleeding
- Blood clots

Any unusual symptoms should be reported to your doctor.[2]

---

[1]Source: www.lungevity.org
[2]Source: www.lungcancer.org

Appendix B

WEBSITES FOR RESOURCES

Disclaimer: These are the websites I found helpful. I do not vouch for their accuracy or endorse products, procedures, services, or medical advice given through these links. Do not substitute my opinion or those found on these websites for those of your personal physician.

ALK Inhibitors

www.alkinhibitors.com
Information on ALK inhibitors

American Cancer Society

www.cancer.org
800-227-2345

Cancer*Care*

www.cancercare.org
www.lungcancer.org
800-813-HOPE (4673)

Clinical Trials

www.clinicaltrials.gov

Cure

www.curetoday.com
Free magazine subscription for cancer survivors and caregivers

Foundation One Medicine

www.foundationmedicine.com
888-988-3639
Performs genomic testing of tumors to determine cancer mutation

GRACE

Global Resource for Advancing Cancer Education
www.cancergrace.org
888-501-1025
Founded by Dr. Howard "Jack" West, President
Thoracic Medical Oncologist at Swedish Cancer Institute

Highlands Oncology Group

www.highlandsoncologygroup.com
479-587-1700

Imerman Angels

www.imermanangels.org
866-IMERMAN (463-7626)
Free personalized one-on-one cancer support for cancer survivors and caregivers

Inspire

www.inspire.com
800-945-0381
Free website to discuss health concerns and treatments with patients/caregivers dealing with patient's exact diagnosis

Lung Cancer Research Foundation

www.lungcancerresearchfoundation.org
212-588-1580

LUNGevity

www.lungevity.org
844-360-5864

MD Anderson Cancer Center

www.mdanderson.org
844-723-1310

National Cancer Institute

www.cancer.gov
800-4-CANCER

Quackwatch

www.quackwatch.org
Exposes health-related frauds, myths, fads, and fallacies for quacky medical treatment

University of Colorado

Denver School of Medicine, Division of Medical Oncology
www.ucdenver.edu/academics/colleges/medicalschool/departments/medicine/medicaloncology

UT Southwestern

www.utswmedicine.org/cancer
214-648-3111

Appendix C

CAREGIVER TIPS

- Make sure the patient's doctors and hospitals are in your insurance plan and treatments are covered.
- Take a list of questions to every appointment. Write down the answers or ask if you may record the appointment. Ask the doctor to explain things in terms you understand.
- Use a free website, such as www.caringbridge.org, to update family and friends.
- Find a support group for the patient *and* caregiver through your church, doctor, hospital, or friends.
- Ask someone to coordinate meals, activities, and errands. Free websites are available: www.lotsahelpinghands.com, www.mealtrain.com, or their Meal Train Plus feature.
- For women with cancer, contact cleaningforareason.org for free periodic cleaning service.
- Find out what disability benefits (including "intermittent" disability) are available through your employer. See if the patient qualifies for Social Security disability.
- Speak with a patient advocate to seek financial assistance.

- Ask if the pharmaceutical company will help pay for any of your travel expenses for out-of-town clinical trials.
- If you are seeking treatment out of town, also find a local doctor for emergencies.
- If you need to travel by air, make sure the doctor approves the patient to fly—in writing if the patient looks sick.
- Angel Flight arranges free air transportation for qualifying medically related needs. Contact www.angelflight.com.
- Make sure the patient has an updated will, a medical power of attorney with a separate HIPAA release authority, a living will (directive to physicians and family), and a durable power of attorney.
- Take care of yourself mentally and physically.
- Give the patient and yourself permission to cry.
- Get a copy of all reports from the doctor, radiology, pathology, and labs, and get a CD of scans and x-rays as soon as they are available. They are usually free.
- Try to understand the terminology on the medical reports.
- Don't assume no news is good news. Follow up. The report may have been overlooked.
- If surgery is needed, ask how long the patient should be off medications that could cause blood clots or prevent blood from clotting.
- Let oral surgeons and dentists know if the patient is taking treatments to strengthen bones prior to an invasive oral procedure.
- If the patient is in a clinical trial, make sure you know what tests and procedures are to be done at each visit and the frequency. Make sure they get properly scheduled.

- Always have a backup plan for everything, including your next treatment option.
- Create a system to organize:
    - Doctors' contact information
    - Account numbers and information to pay bills online if you get stuck out of town at a hospital
    - List of medications (including chemo) with dosage, contraindications, and dates started and stopped
    - Daily journal to log health problems, symptoms, improvements, weight, oxygen, heart rate, blood pressure, etc.
    - Procedure instructions for CT scan, MRI, PET, etc.
    - Questions to ask doctors and their answers
    - Treatment summary—date, doctor/facility, procedure, surgery, diagnosis, medication prescribed, dosage
    - Contact information for people who offered to help and what help they offered
    - Hotel information in the area of your treatment
    - Maps of the area and facility where the treatment is received
    - Treatment options
    - Pamphlets on the treatment received
    - Medication information (instructions and side effects)
    - Nutritionist information
    - Appointments
    - Explanation of benefits (EOBs)
    - Lab results
    - Pathology reports
    - Patient reports from doctors
    - Radiology reports and CDs
    - Clinical trial information

- If you have problems with insurance or facilities, write down the name of the person you spoke with, the date, the time, and what was said.
- Keep a spreadsheet for medical expenses. Keep track of the dates doctors were seen, as well as what tests and procedures were performed, and match them up with the EOBs to ensure you aren't billed in error. Document when expenses were paid to avoid duplicate payments. Follow up if you're due a refund.
- If you have cancer insurance, know what reimbursements you are entitled to and make sure they pay you the proper amount.
- Keep your car filled with enough gas to get to medical appointments or to the hospital in an emergency. Keep it maintained with regular oil changes and tire rotations.
- Keep a checklist of things to take to the emergency room. Don't forget your cell phone charger.
- Keep luggage prepacked with basics for frequent trips to the ER.
- If you go to the ER, take a summary report of the treatment history, the most recent doctors' and radiologists' reports, and a CD of the most recent scans.
- Take the patient's medication bottles with you to the ER, especially if you have a specialty drug.
- Take the *caregiver's* medication bottles with you to the ER in case you end up staying at the hospital.
- Sanitize items in hotel and hospital rooms: TV remote, food tray, light switches, phone, keyboard, etc.
- In the hospital, write down all medications given to the patient (ask the nurse what they are and to spell them for you), the time, the dosage, and what they're for.

- Leave a spare house key with a trusted neighbor or family member. Have them check on your home periodically during lengthy trips.
- Discuss funeral plans and make arrangements before the need arises.
- Learn how to pay the family bills, reconcile a bank statement, where to file or find important paperwork, and where to find passwords to all accounts, including social media accounts.
- Ask what food, drink, or activity the patient should avoid on medications.
- Find out if it's safe to have sexual relations without protection while on chemo, since some drugs are excreted in bodily fluids.
- Find out if it's safe to get pregnant while being treated.
- Ask for medications to deal with side effects.
- Seek treatment for depression, if needed.
- It's a patient's right to have full disclosure to make an informed decision.
- It's a patient's right to refuse treatment.
- You are your own best advocate. Be vigilant. Even the best professionals don't know everything and can make mistakes.

To see Chris Haga's journey through his own eyes,
read his companion book:

Cancer on Two Wheels
A Spiritual Journey with Stage IV Lung Cancer

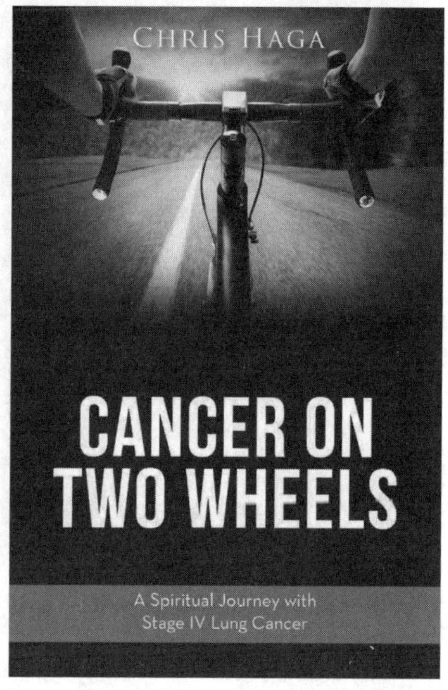

About the Author

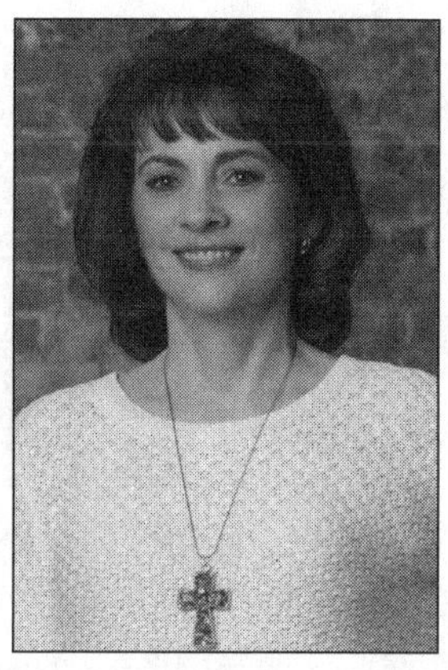

DeLayne Haga graduated from Oklahoma State University with a Bachelor of Science in Business Administration and has owned a secretarial/bookkeeping business since 1997. DeLayne and Chris, her husband of thirty-two years, raised two sons. Her hobbies include reading, gardening, baking sweets, and documenting the family's memories through photographs.

After her husband was diagnosed with cancer, DeLayne mentored caregivers of lung cancer survivors. She was a member of the Cancer Encouragement Group at her church and helped form a support group for caregivers. Following Chris's death, she became involved with the Widows' Encouragement Group, the Soul Care Ministry, and the Widows' Ministry advisory committee at her church. Seeing a need for younger widows to have an opportunity to socialize with other widows, she helped form a group for young, active widows in and around her community.

Residing in McKinney, Texas, DeLayne is rekindling old friendships, making new friends, and continuing to trust God to provide for her needs and guide her in the next chapter of her life.